AF333850

Updates in Surgery

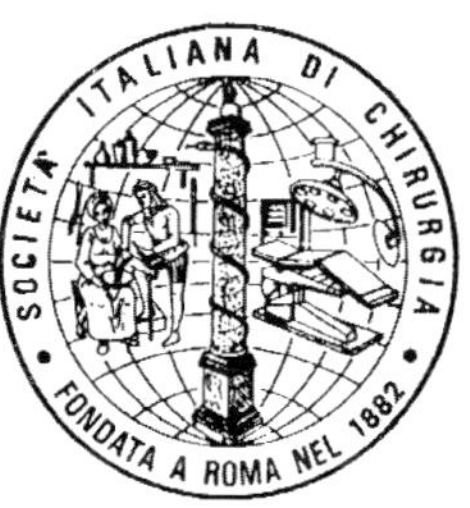

Antonio Bolognese • Luciano Izzo

Surgery in Multimodal Management of Solid Tumors

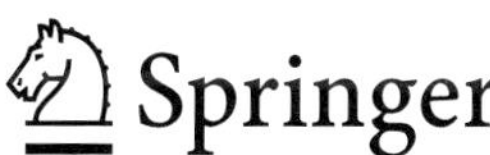 Springer

Antonio Bolognese
Department of Surgery "Pietro Valdoni"
Policlinico Umberto I
La Sapienza University
Rome, Italy

Luciano Izzo
Department of Surgery "Pietro Valdoni"
Policlinico Umberto I
La Sapienza University
Rome, Italy

The publication and the distribution of this volume have been supported by the Italian Society of Surgery

Library of Congress Control Number: 2008936504

ISBN 978-88-470-1084-0 Springer Milan Berlin Heidelberg New York
e-ISBN 978-88-470-1085-7

Springer is a part of Springer Science+Business Media
springer.com
© Springer-Verlag Italia 2009

Cover design: Simona Colombo,Milan, Italy
Typesetting: Graphostudio, Milan, Italy
Printing and binding: Arti Grafiche Nidasio, Assago, Italy

Printed in Italy
Springer-Verlag Italia S.r.l. – Via Decembrio 28 – I-20137 Milan

Foreword

The contributions of science and technology are essential to sound clinical practice, as they enable a clear assessment of the clinical manifestations of disease and, in turn, form the basis for the appropriate medical or surgical treatment.

There are two major parts to this volume. In the first, the relationship between cancer biology and surgery and the challenges posed by the one on the other are discussed. In the second, the contributions of biochemistry, physiology, pathology, imaging, chemotherapy, radiation therapy and surgery to the diagnosis and management of solid tumors are considered. The information is addressed not only to experienced surgeons but also to those entering or still in training.

I wish to thank the distinguished specialists who have contributed to this book. Their efforts have resulted in a comprehensive review of the state-of-the-art knowledge regarding multimodal treatment of solid tumors.

Rome, October 2008

Roberto Tersigni
President, Italian Society of Surgery

Foreword

It was 1968 when Prof. Paolo Biocca, appointed by Prof. Pietro Valdoni as a reference point of the School, had just been called by the Faculty of Medicine and Surgery of 'La Sapienza' University of Rome to hold the Professorship of Special Surgical Pathology.

As was rarely the case, although I was one of his closest pupils, Prof. Biocca called for me, and after having politely knocked on the door, I entered his office and saw before me a gentleman whom Prof. Biocca introduced as a colleague who was accompanying his newly graduated son. As was the custom then, this young man was assigned to me so that I could be his tutor.

From that day on, Antonio Bolognese and I have been sharing the life of a University Institute of Surgery according to the rules of that time – with joy and grief, but also with the absolute dedication and enthusiasm of those who had chosen to become surgeons. I undertook my commitment very seriously, in part because ten years earlier my surgeon-father had assigned me to Prof. Biocca, first in Cagliari and then in Catania.

This premise was necessary, because these elements define the concepts of the School in which we have lived and for which we have made great sacrifices.

So began Antonio Bolognese his training, with a scrupulous educational commitment to research and assistance. His great intellectual honesty and commitment have been fundamental in his maturity and have led him to fulfill a brilliant career.

His interests have always focused on the oncologic field where his wide views as a cultured surgeon always attentive to the evolution of science have led him to collaborate with prestigious international institutions with which he has built intense and profitable cultural exchanges.

Oncologic surgery has become an increasingly interdisciplinary field, open to equal collaboration among complementary disciplines such as diagnostics, medical oncology, radiotherapy and more recently, genetics. The work which is presented in this volume is therefore the result of a measured, conscious development of the problems of oncologic surgery by those who have come a long way, but which is projected into a future where everything must contribute to improving the prognosis of patients no longer abandoned to their uncertain destiny with little hope of improvement.

Today, Prof. Bolognese provides us with comfort by underlining that the joint commitment of different medical fields, each respectful of the different cultures and each humbly willing to welcome and blend their different therapeutic potentialities, is the main road for achieving progress in oncologic surgery.

This is the message I have gleaned from in this volume, and for this I thank Prof. Bolognese on behalf of everybody, and wish him to continue his endeavors in this field in which he truly believes.

Vincenzo Stipa
Professor of General Surgery,
La Sapienza University, Rome

Preface

My sincere and heartfelt thanks to the President and to the Board of Directors of the Italian Society of Surgery for having assigned me the task of compiling this report on "Surgery in Multimodal Management of Solid Tumors".

In a time when the most recent epidemiologic research indicates an increase of about 50% in cancer over the next 10 years, surgery continues to be the most efficacious treatment of solid tumors in terms of recovery, while its combination with other treatments improves survival curves especially in the advanced forms.

It was therefore with profound enthusiasm that I accepted the task entrusted to me because I deem it useful to be able to provide my colleagues and readers with the opportunity of approaching one of the most up-to-date and complex issues of our professional practice. I also accepted this invitation with a similar degree of apprehension, being aware of the difficulties in carrying out such a daunting task while fulfilling the expectations implied by it.

This is why, while compiling this report, I felt the need to ask for the contribution of some prestigious friends, all experts in their relative fields, and especially the involvement of many colleagues of the "Pietro Valdoni" Department of Surgery and of La Sapienza University of Rome, an institution constantly at the forefront in the national and international field of the study and treatment of tumors, an institution in which I was fortunate enough to receive my training and of which I am honored to be a part.

The aim of my task first of all has been to provide readers with both the current and constantly evolving pathophysiologic knowledge required for building the foundation of a specific education enabling surgeons to meet the fundamental targets in surgical oncology. Secondly, this volume aims to present an update on the real possibilities offered by the cooperation between surgeon and pathologist and by chemotherapy, radiotherapy and gene therapy in the treatment of tumors in the light of the most recent scientific achievements. Lastly, the report presents the experiences and cases drawn mostly from our School regarding some of the major issues in oncologic surgery.

This overview does not pretend to elucidate or to summarize all aspects of oncologic surgery, but rather to be the result of a general consideration on cancer surgery, on its rational bases, on its interaction with other treatment modalities, on its desirable and expected developments and on its probable future evolution.

Lastly, I wish to extend my affectionate thanks to Prof. Vincenzo Stipa for having provided me the opportunity of undertaking the path of my education, both as man and surgeon, for allowing me to be constantly by his side, capturing the essence of what can be fundamental for achieving the necessary balance for carrying out such a burdensome, delicate and fascinating professional practice – the practice of a University professor of surgery.

Antonio Bolognese

Contents

Contributors

Fabio Accarpio
Department of Surgery "P. Valdoni", University of Rome "La Sapienza", Azienda Policlinico Umberto I, Rome, Italy

Anna Maria Baccheschi
Department of Surgery "P. Valdoni", University of Rome "La Sapienza", Azienda Policlinico Umberto I, Rome, Italy

Genoveffa Balducci
University of Rome "La Sapienza", II Faculty of Medicine, UOC Chirurgia A, Sant'Andrea Hospital, Rome, Italy

Giuliano Barugola
Department of Surgery, Policlinico "GB Rossi", Verona, Italy

Claudio Bassi
Department of Surgery, Policlinico "GB Rossi", Verona, Italy

Francesca Berardi
University of Rome "La Sapienza", II Faculty of Medicine, UOC Chirurgia A, Sant'Andrea Hospital, Rome, Italy

Daniele Biacchi
Department of Surgery "P. Valdoni", University of Rome "La Sapienza", Azienda Policlinico Umberto I, Rome, Italy

Antonio Bolognese
Department of Surgery "P. Valdoni", University of Rome "La Sapienza", Azienda Policlinico Umberto I, Rome, Italy

Francesco Borrini
"Belcolle" Hospital, Viterbo - Department of Surgery "P. Valdoni", University of Rome "La Sapienza", Azienda Policlinico Umberto I, Rome, Italy

Vincenzo Cangemi
Department of Surgery "P. Valdoni", University of Rome "La Sapienza", Azienda
Policlinico Umberto I, Rome, Italy

Linda Cerbone
Department of Experimental Medicine, University of Rome "La Sapienza",
Azienda Policlinico Umberto I, Rome, Italy

Tommaso Cornali
Department of Surgery "P. Valdoni", University of Rome "La Sapienza", Azienda
Policlinico Umberto I, Rome, Italy

Alessandro Crocetti
Department of Surgery "P. Valdoni", University of Rome "La Sapienza", Azienda
Policlinico Umberto I, Rome, Italy

Pierfrancesco Di Cello
Department of Surgery "P. Valdoni", University of Rome "La Sapienza", Azienda
Policlinico Umberto I, Rome, Italy

Angelo Di Giorgio
Department of Surgery "P. Valdoni", University of Rome "La Sapienza", Azienda
Policlinico Umberto I, Rome, Italy

Marisa Di Seri
Department of Experimental Medicine, University of Rome "La Sapienza",
Azienda Policlinico Umberto I, Rome, Italy

Dominique Elias
Department of Surgical Oncology, "Gustave-Roussy" Institute, Villejuif, France

Massimo Falconi
Department of Surgery, Policlinico "GB Rossi", Verona, Italy

Silvia I.S. Fattoruso
Istituto Nazionale Tumori "Regina Elena", Rome, Italy

Silvia Femia
Department of Surgery "P. Valdoni", University of Rome "La Sapienza", Azienda
Policlinico Umberto I, Rome, Italy

Enrico Fiori
Department of Surgery "P. Valdoni", University of Rome "La Sapienza", Azienda
Policlinico Umberto I, Rome, Italy

Sergio Gazzanelli
Department of Anaestesiology and Intensive Care, University of Rome "La Sapienza", Azienda Policlinico Umberto I, Rome, Italy

Laura Giacinti
"San Giuseppe" Hospital, Albano Laziale (Rome), Italy

Alberto Gulino
Department of Experimental Medicine, University of Rome "La Sapienza", Azienda Policlinico Umberto I, Rome, Italy

Clemente Iascone
Department of Surgery "P. Valdoni", University of Rome "La Sapienza", Azienda Policlinico Umberto I, Rome, Italy

Luciano Izzo
Department of Surgery "P. Valdoni", University of Rome "La Sapienza", Azienda Policlinico Umberto I, Rome, Italy

Massimo Lopez
Istituto Nazionale Tumori "Regina Elena", Rome, Italy

Giuseppe Malleo
Department of Surgery, Policlinico "GB Rossi", Verona, Italy

Riccardo Maurizi Enrici
University of Rome "La Sapienza", II Faculty of Medicine, UOC Chirurgia A, Sant'Andrea Hospital, Rome, Italy

Paolo Meloni
Department of Surgery "P. Valdoni", University of Rome "La Sapienza", Azienda Policlinico Umberto I, Rome, Italy

Paolo Mercantini
University of Rome "La Sapienza", II Faculty of Medicine, UOC Chirurgia A, Sant'Andrea Hospital, Rome, Italy

Pietro L. Mingazzini
University of Rome "La Sapienza", Azienda Policlinico Umberto I, Rome, Italy

Mattia F. Osti
University of Rome "La Sapienza", II Faculty of Medicine, UOC Chirurgia A, Sant'Andrea Hospital, Rome, Italy

Annalisa Paliotta
Department of Surgery "P. Valdoni", University of Rome "La Sapienza", Azienda
Policlinico Umberto I, Rome, Italy

Paolo Pederzoli
Department of Surgery, Policlinico "GB Rossi", Verona, Italy

Niccolò Petrucciani
University of Rome "La Sapienza", II Faculty of Medicine, UOC Chirurgia A,
Sant'Andrea Hospital, Rome, Italy

Dario Pietrasanta
Department of Surgery "P. Valdoni", University of Rome "La Sapienza", Azienda
Policlinico Umberto I, Rome, Italy

Federica Pulcini
Department of Surgery "P. Valdoni", University of Rome "La Sapienza", Azienda
Policlinico Umberto I, Rome, Italy

Francesca Ricci
Department of Surgery "P. Valdoni", University of Rome "La Sapienza", Azienda
Policlinico Umberto I, Rome, Italy

Paolo Sammartino
Department of Surgery "P. Valdoni", University of Rome "La Sapienza", Azienda
Policlinico Umberto I, Rome, Italy

Simone Sibio
Department of Surgery "P. Valdoni", University of Rome "La Sapienza", Azienda
Policlinico Umberto I, Rome, Italy

Silvia Trombetta
Department of Surgery "P. Valdoni", University of Rome "La Sapienza", Azienda
Policlinico Umberto I, Rome, Italy

Fabio Zarantonello
Department of Surgery, Policlinico "GB Rossi", Verona, Italy

Vincenzo Ziparo
University of Rome "La Sapienza", II Faculty of Medicine, UOC Chirurgia A,
Sant'Andrea Hospital, Rome, Italy

Introduction

Surgery was the first and for many years the only therapeutic modality of solid tumors, even though over the past few decades, randomized studies and meta-analyses have demonstrated the advantages of combined treatment in a large variety of tumors in which prolongation of survival has been attained.

Improved knowledge of the natural history of tumors, together with the technical and technologic advancements in diagnostics and in other disciplines, such as radiotherapy, medical oncology, biology, pathologic anatomy, immunology and genetics, have modified the treatment of many tumors and urge surgeons to question the role of surgical radicality, especially in cases of advanced tumor, at a time when cancer is often related to genetic modifications, whose nature and extent we are trying to manipulate.

The correct approach to multidisciplinary therapies, the timing of treatment to be performed in combination or in succession, the planning of interdisciplinary studies and research, the problem of the resection margins also in relation to histologic type and to the biologic aggressiveness of tumors, are currently essential conditions for an adequate surgical operation, according to current oncologic standards. Today, the oncologist surgeon must therefore be a specialist with deep multidisciplinary knowledge and with the awareness of the therapeutic potentialities of combined treatment.

Even though surgery continues to be the main therapeutic method for most solid tumors, the results obtained with surgery alone, especially in the advanced stages, but where the tumor is still operable, are conditioned by the reoccurrence of disease, sometimes in a local-regional area, sometimes distant. In these cases, the failure of surgical treatment is due to the fact that the cancer, at the time of diagnosis already has a microscopic extension that goes beyond the resection margins or a systemic diffusion that cannot be detected with the means currently available.

In order to reduce the number of relapses and improve curability, other local-regional treatment modalities were added to surgery, such as radiotherapy, or systemic treatment such as chemo- or immunotherapy. The efficacy of these treatment modalities denominated "adjuvant" has been demonstrated in controlled studies in various types of tumor.

A. Bolognese, L. Izzo (eds.), *Surgery in Multimodal Management of Solid Tumors.*
©Springer-Verlag Italia 2009

A second target of combined treatments is sometimes the preservation of an anatomic part or a function; in this way surgery is less radical and more respectful of organ function, combining radio- and chemotherapy to surgery. The therapeutic combinations, which in these cases are defined "neo-adjuvant", represent a rapid and constant evolving aspect of oncologic surgery and increasingly define the borders between oncologic surgery and general surgery.

Cancer therapy is therefore becoming increasingly complex and today many solid tumors, even in the initial stages, are treated with more than one therapeutic modality. Consequently, this multidisciplinary approach requires the coordination and the consent of several specialists.

The oncologist radiotherapist provides an important local and local-regional treatment technique for cancer, more and more frequently combined with the simultaneous administration of chemotherapy. The oncologist physician has the task of administering and monitoring the chemotherapy, the hormone therapy and in some cases the biologic therapy. The oncologist surgeon, lastly, is becoming a "specialist" who treats neoplasms with increasingly standardized and precise surgical techniques, who must have particular skills that complete those usually required by specialists of organ surgery, with a strong aptitude for collective decisions.

Part 1
General Principles

Chapter 1
Surgery and Tumors

Antonio Bolognese, Dominique Elias

Surgery is the fundamental treatment option in most solid tumors, but it is no longer the sole therapeutic weapon available. Instead it needs to be integrated in a considerably more complex multidisciplinary strategy, with two main aims:
- To guarantee recovery and increase the duration of survival through the control of the disease, not only at the local-regional level, but also in general
- To guarantee good quality of life by means of the most conservative possible treatment which maintains organ function and a good image of the organism

In such a complex scenario, the foremost role of surgery – prevention, diagnosis and control of the disease – remains unchanged. Oncologic surgery has never been included in the various specialties with its own autonomy, for logical reasons considering that multiple and different organs may be involved, in emergency and non-emergency situations, with the intent at times curative, at times palliative. It is however taught in many specialties, although its fundamental principles are either little divulged or are based on knowledge which is rapidly made obsolete by scientific progress.

Oncologic surgery can be currently interpreted as a quite peculiar specialty requiring particular skills which complement those required in other specialties. Therefore it seems indispensable to analyze and discuss some of the fundamental mechanisms of the interaction of surgery with tumor growth in light of the most recent knowledge of oncologic physiopathology.

It is known that the diffusion of neoplastic cells is an early and constant event at the time the primitive tumor infiltrates the submucosa, overpassing the basal membrane and invading the interstitial stroma: the host's immune potency, however, can modify tumor progression in such a way as to inhibit or facilitate it by giving rise to bleeding, lymph diffusion or spread by contiguity with local organs.

Hematogenous Diffusion

Hematogenous diffusion has been highlighted since 1965 and is a constant occurrence starting from peri-tumoral veins. Tumoral manipulation and pre-sur-

A. Bolognese, L. Izzo (eds.), *Surgery in Multimodal Management of Solid Tumors.*
©Springer-Verlag Italia 2009

gery biological perturbations may significantly increase the diffusion of tumor cells [1]. Salsbury demonstrated that after ligature of the inferior mesenteric artery in patients undergoing surgery for colorectal cancer, the presence of neoplastic cells in the peripheral blood was positive in 60% of the cases versus 10% prior to ligature [2]. Preventive ligature of all vascular peduncles is not performed in all cases and controlled prospective trials have shown no significant variations in terms of survival in patients with preventive ligature compared to a control group; these considerations therefore put into perspective the classic dogma of preventive ligature of vascular peduncles in oncologic surgery [1–3].

A quantification of hematogenous diffusion was performed in man in 1988. The number of tumor cells penetrating the renal vein of kidney-cancer patients with a tumor diameter ranging from 6 to 8 cm is between 2.3 and 5 billion within 24 hours [4]; this is a considerable number which increases with increasing tumor size.

The detection of tumor cells circulating in the blood has be analyzed in numerous studies over the past few years, thus clearly showing that these cells represent the origin of the metastatic process [5]. It has been demonstrated, though, that the presence of circulating tumor cells does not always result in metastasis, given the metastatic inefficacy of some cells, since only some clones can result in metastasis and some are eliminated by the host's immune defenses.

Recently it has been demonstrated that not all circulating tumor cells are genetically identical. This genetic heterogeneity is particularly evident in cells from the primitive tumor (unstable genome) and less so in those from metastasis (stable genome) [6]. This represents a major problem for chemotherapy or gene therapy.

Lymphatic Diffusion

Lymphatic diffusion of tumors is one of the major problems in oncologic surgery, being significantly correlated to the accuracy of detection methods: it is an early and quite constant event. Diffusion follows the less resistant paths through the follicles and thin-wall capillaries. Lymph glands are not very effective filters for tumor cells: most cells simply pass through them without being trapped and enter the blood stream. The inoculation of tumor cells marked with radioactive substances with a different nature and different size into the adjacent lymph node vessels shows that only 13% of them are filtered by the lymph nodes [7]: in contrast, lymphatic infiltration is frequent.

The lymphophilic character of tumors varies depending on the histological type of the tumor: it is weak for tumors such as clear cell sarcomas and carcinomas of the kidney, while it is marked for adenocarcinomas of the digestive system and breast. In 1991, Isono demonstrated that lymph node involvement depends on the degree of tumor infiltration, underlining that 30% of epidermoid carcinomas of the esophagus infiltrating the muscolaris mucosae results in lymph node metastasis and this figure rises to 52% when the submucosa is also infiltrated [8].

The evaluation of lymphatic diffusion also depends on the number of lymph nodes that the surgeon provides to the pathologist and on the type of method used for the detection. Hermaneck has demonstrated that in the case of colorectal carcinoma, as the number of lymph nodes examined increases, the chances of detecting a higher number of lymph nodes invaded also increases [9]. For this reason the 1997 UICC classification already took into consideration the minimum number of lymph nodes to be examined in relation to the site of the primary tumor, in order to define the lymphatic invasion with precision [10].

With regard to the study of lymph nodes, it has now become clear that the more and better they are tested, the more their infiltration is observed, which is important for the diagnosis of most tumors [11].

By completely dissolving the fat tissue, the "clearing technique" assists in the identification and examination of lymph nodes with 1-5 mm diameter which otherwise would not be assessable [12], with positive findings increasing from 20 to 50%. This technique is nonetheless very complex, expensive and requires more than 10 days to complete [13].

In 1994 Greenson demonstrated that by means of immunohistochemistry and the use of anti-cytokeratin antibodies neoplastic cells can be detected in 28% of the cases previously classified as negative with traditional methods. The prognostic value of the detection of lymph node metastasis is made evident in the fact that 5-year mortality rises from 3% of the N- cases to 43% in the N+ cases. The author also underlines that in this way, cases classified Dukes B, with the detection of metastasis previously undetected, can be re-classified Dukes C and so they can be included in adjuvant chemotherapy protocols with an improvement in survival [14].

In 1995 Hayashi studied 120 patients with Dukes B colorectal cancer using the PCR (Protein Chain Reaction) technique, looking for mutations of K-ras and p53 genes. Such mutations have been seen in 60% of patients; 73% of them, after 5 years, presented a local relapse versus 0% of patients who had no mutation in the genes examined. Therefore PCR and RT-PCR seem to be methods capable of identifying cells which express tumor markers otherwise undetectable in patients with localized or metastatic tumor and can represent a valid instrument of study of the biology of metastases [15, 16].

These investigation methods, while sophisticated and perhaps not feasible in all centers, can be used to detect the presence of micrometastases and to more precisely evaluate the stage of the disease, with consequent optimization of therapeutic protocols.

The importance of the identification of micrometastases in lymph nodes and of isolated tumor cells as factors that can impact the diagnosis has been documented by the inclusion of the last TNM classification of 2002 of the abbreviations "i" and "mol" (immunohistochemistry and molecular biology) beside to the N and M parameter (American Joint Committee on Cancer – sixth edition).

Marrow Infiltration

Another question which has aroused much interest is the presence of tumor cells in the bone marrow. In 1992, Lindeman published a study on 88 patients with colorectal cancer using anti-cytokeratin CK18 monoclonal antibodies for the detection of neoplastic cells: 32% of patients turned out to be positive of whom 57% developed metastases versus 30% of those turned out to be negative [17].

Marrow infiltration is seen globally in 35–60% of cases, it has a prognostic value, but its demonstration depends on the means used. These cells behave as "dormant" cells, since 90% of them are in G0 stage and only 10% of them express the K67 proliferation marker [18, 19].

Local Implants of Tumor Cells

A particular occurrence specific to oncologic surgery is the possible tumor dissemination in the surgical field. This event is a highly developing process, characterized by simple biological mechanisms which occur even if the surgeon does not directly manipulate the tumor: the opening of veins and lymph vessels containing the tumor cells is the cause of the event and cell dissemination is observed in the blood collected in the surgical field [20].

Dissemination and local implant of neoplastic cells usually occurs most frequently after spontaneous perforation of the tumor, after its rupture for biopsy or exeresis purposes or when a tumor is visible under the serosa. These considerations explain, in part, the onset of local relapses after surgery and the importance of performing an exsanguinate operation also limiting the lymphorrhagia. Neoplastic cells in fact become trapped in fibrin deposits which rapidly cover the wound areas and have a specific affinity for normal pre-surgery fibrinous adhesions, which are seen as early as 30 minutes after surgery: cells adhere to them due to the rich presence of arginine-glycine-aspartate (RDG) tripeptide complex through integrines which are numerous on their membrane [21].

Tumor cells entrapped in the fibrin in this way are in a sort of "sanctuary" where they cannot be attacked by any drug through the systemic route because of a lack of neovascularization and in which they find a fertile territory for growth [22].

Understanding of these mechanisms has contributed to the development of strategies aimed at avoiding the taking of tumor cells and the therapy of peritoneal carcinosis according to Sugarbaker's concepts.

Consequences of Surgery on the Immune Status and Neoplastic Growth

A particular event of oncologic surgery, considered particularly important in recent times, is the repercussion that the surgical operation can have on tumor growth and patient immune status. In some cases of advanced cancer there would appear little rationale for the use of "local" treatment such as surgery, although good results can be obtained. One example is the surgical exeresis of liver metastasis of colorectal origin which can "cure" a third of the patients who can benefit from it [23]. No other treatment reaches such results and therefore it can be concluded that surgery alone can "cure" some metastatic tumors.

The effectiveness of surgery is even more remarkable if one considers that during the surgical and post-surgical period it is accompanied by negative modifications: considerable increase in tumor-cell dissemination via hematogenous route [24], immunodepression lasting about seven days [25, 26], worsened by blood transfusions with facilitation of the taking and growth of TGF and EGF tumor cells [27].

This is why efforts are underway to use immunotherapy to reduce the negative effects surgery causes to the patient's immune system. In this regard, a randomized study performed by Elias on patients undergoing resection for liver metastasis showed that the control group was immunodepressed while preoperative five-day interleukin-2 reversed postoperative immunodepression in the study group [26, 28]. It remains to be demonstrated what the impact of such preoperative immunostimulation will be on survival: a randomized study compared the evolution of 69 patients treated or not with subcutaneous interleukin-2 during gastrectomy for cancer, with the results demonstrating that the treated group showed a fivefold reduction in postoperative complications and a longer survival rate ($p = 0.06$) [29].

Surgery is often defined "radical" meaning the total removal of the disease which can be seen macroscopically; it would, instead, be more correct to define it "tumor reduction" surgery, since it fails to remove a portion of tumor cells such as the circulating cells, the marrow dormant cells and the already existent micrometastases. In fact, the reduction of a tumoral mass from 1 kg to 1 g reduces the number of tumor cells only from 10^{12} to 10^{9} [30].

Nevertheless, even taking into account its incomplete character and its negative effects, surgery remains a considerably effective treatment and, if combined with other therapies, it can offer better results in terms of reduction of local relapses and improvement of the survival curves, especially in advanced tumors.

It appears more and more evident, however, that multiple chemotherapeutic treatments are more effective depending on the reduction of the tumor volume. It is certainly in the adjuvant treatment after surgery and when the residual disease can no longer be demonstrated by imaging radiology or laboratory tests that chemotherapy undoubtedly increases the recovery rate: the addition of folfox after resection of third-stage stomach cancer reduces relapse formation by 23% [31] compared to 5-fluoride-uracil alone which already reduced the risk by 41% in relation to the lack of adjuvant chemotherapy [32].

It is therefore legitimate to state a simple yet fundamental therapeutic concept: surgery which removes the macroscopic disease, combined with adjuvant chemotherapy to treat the residual disease offers the highest healing possibilities to patients.

This principle is the basis of treatment for some peritoneal carcinomas through surgical exeresis of all the metastases with a size of a few millimeters, in combination with immediate intraoperative chemo-hyperthermia, aimed at eradicating the residual metastases with a size not exceeding 1 cm [33]: this treatment is in fact still proving its effectiveness [34, 35].

The prognostic impact of chemotherapy, combined with surgery, seems equally clear in a study by Adam [36] which shows that in patients undergoing hepatectomy for at least four metastases of colic origin, 5-year survival is 34% in patients who were stable under chemotherapy, while it decreased to 8% in patients who had a progression of the disease: it would therefore be logical to conclude that this type of hepatectomy should be no longer proposed to this kind of patient.

In this therapeutic combination the role of chemotherapy is as important as the role of surgery, but in this setting it is fundamental that the effectiveness of chemotherapy be preliminarily tested. In the near future it is likely that functional imaging diagnostics (PET-Scan, study of tumor vascularization with 3D ultrasound with contrast material prior to chemotherapy) will provide this important information. Another controversial topic is the surgical indication to resect a nonsymptomatic primary tumor when there is also metastasis. The debate is becoming more and more interesting with the increasing effectiveness of multiple chemotherapy. Traditionally, the exeresis of the primary tumor is considered a categorical imperative both for patient comfort and for oncologic reasons (the primary tumor would spread more than metastases). Instead, a recent comparative study performed on 12 patients with liver metastasis (6 of whom were operated for the removal of a primary colon tumor) demonstrated that tumor resection is oncologically deleterious: in fact a significant increase in PET activity was demonstrated in the metastases left in situ only in the group of patients who underwent colectomy with a concurrent significant fall in circulating endostatin and angiostatin, which are endogenous inhibitors of angiogenesis. This seems to suggest that the primary tumor secretes angiogenesis-inhibiting substances, and its exeresis removed this constraint thus favoring the growth of metastases [37]. Furthermore, with regard to the timing of therapeutic combinations aimed at improving survival, the rational bases of the concept to combine chemotherapy or pre-surgical immunotherapy are sufficiently clear: it has in fact been demonstrated that surgery is a moment of stress and immune weakness, with a higher possibility of tumor spread. These two occurrences combine to create a high-risk period, and such occurrence, which can be easily demonstrated with experimental models, have been known since 1910 [4, 38]. In the mouse operated for breast cancer, the preoperative injection of 10 mg/kg of doxorubicin produces 92% survival at 3 weeks, versus only 23% in the control group. Moreover, if the drug is injected four days after surgery, survival is 38% compared with 70% if doxorubicin is injected four days prior to surgery [39]. In female patients it has been observed that the injection of cyclophosphamide on the first and fifth day postmastectomy for cancer increases 5-year survival by 10% [40]. It is indeed amazing remarkable to see how pre-surgical chemotherapy has only had limited use;

perhaps this is due to the fact that for a long time chemotherapy was thought to cause alterations in the wound healing processes, and to increase postoperative infections and specific complications. Therefore, high dose chemotherapy should be administered with fewer concerns both prior to and during surgery. Perhaps its impact needs to be demonstrated with a randomized trial. In this light Elias has been claiming and demonstrating since 1987 that patients who have undergone hepatectomy for metastasis can be treated with postoperative intraportal chemotherapy immediately and for the subsequent 14 days [28], and that over the past 8 years in 200 patients having undergone surgery for peritoneal carcinosis of colorectal origin – a major operation combined with intraperitoneal chemohyperthermia with high dose drugs – the results are more than satisfactory [41, 42].

Efficacy of Oncologic Surgery

It is reasonably safe to state that in terms of recovery surgery alone is the most effective treatment against cancer in the therapy of solid tumors, especially in those cases where truly effective chemotherapy is not always feasible, such as melanomas, sarcomas, or adenocarcinomas of pancreas and kidneys.

Surgical resection is just one of the treatment options for these increasingly numerous chemosensitive tumors. This is the case of colorectal, esophageal and ovarian tumors, in which the therapeutic schemes increasingly use neoadjuvant chemotherapy as primary treatment and surgery as an adjuvant treatment. In this case the therapeutic combination definitely offers better results for the reduction of local relapses and the improvement of survival curves, especially in advanced cancer, and systemic treatment plays a fundamental role, similar to surgical treatment.

In this setting in particular the presence of metastases in different sites loses its prognostic value, as long as surgery is able to remove them completely with curative intent: at this point the total number of assessable and resectable metastases becomes preponderant for prognosis purposes [43]. The role of surgery also undergoes constant change, both according to the progress of the systemic treatments and to its specific limitations: it is no rare event, in fact, in case of a very effective or long-lasting neoadjuvant therapy that imaging diagnostics demonstrates the disappearance of liver or pulmonary metastases of small size. It is unlikely that these metastases have been totally destroyed by chemotherapy, and so in these cases we might either expect them to reappear after the interruption of chemotherapy and then treat them surgically, or we may decide to resect the entire areas where they were located (with the risk of resecting too much or too little tissue). The decision is even more complex when only a part of these metastases reoccurs: the addition of aggressive local-regional chemotherapy with intra-arterial oxaliplatin for metastases of colic origin has demonstrated that their disappearance at diagnostic imaging studies for more than four months meant "sterilization" in about 70% of cases [44].

Surgery instead plays a secondary role in tumors with a high chemosensitivity, e.g. testicular tumors and pediatric tumors. In non-seminoma testicular cancer, in fact, the removal of lymph-node, liver or pulmonary metastases, after normalization or almost normalization of the tumor marker values, reveals necrosis in 60% of cases, teratoma in 35%, and neoplastic activity in only 15% of the cases.

In terms of cost/benefit ratio, surgery remains at present the fundamental fulcrum of solid tumor therapy, and continues to progress orienting its own development in different directions: minimalist and maximalist trend, multidisciplinary therapeutic combination, modification of the therapeutic timing, utilization of modifiers of biological responses, standardization of treatments [45].

In particular, oncologic surgery, as far as orientation is concerned, is in many situations more conservative, thanks to the more precise knowledge of prognosis, the more appropriate choice of the type of operation modulated based on the stage of the tumor and the effectiveness of the multidisciplinary combined therapies.

In some cases, however, the limited effectiveness of neo- and/or adjuvant therapies, especially in advanced tumors, and the more accurate knowledge of the natural history and of the stage, require considerably more radical interventions, sustained, moreover, by progress in the techniques of anesthesiology and resuscitation. Therefore, extensive lymphadenectomies, synchronous exeresis of liver and pulmonary metastases can be performed, as well as simultaneous multidisciplinary treatments for peritoneal carcinosis [8, 22].

The Future of Oncologic Surgery

Tumor surgery will undergo change in the future, just as it has undergone change in the past. Progress will undoubtedly be correlated with the development of the techniques of biology, of pathologic anatomy, of imaging diagnostics and with the development of genomics and proteinomics.

Research carried out on "micrometastases" have recently acquired particular importance and have aroused interest, enthusiasm, but also some doubt. Interest and enthusiasm have been shown for the development of increasingly reliable detection methods, whereas doubt is related to the role that the detection of micrometastases in lymph nodes, the bone marrow and the circulating blood can have on prognosis and, consequently, on the choice and timing of the combined treatments, in order to improve survival [15].

As for the utilization of some substances capable of modifying the biologic response, currently a natural noxious biologic process can be inhibited, or in contrast can stimulate a favorable physiologic event [46]. Some ongoing clinical trials, although in a preliminary phase, have in fact demonstrated the important role of neoangiogenesis on the tumor growth. These trials, which use some inhibitors of neoangiogenesis (cetuximab, bevacizumab, etc.), have shown the absence of pharmacologic resistance despite the long-term treatment, a high grade of specificity and a reduction of side-effects, with increasingly encouraging long-term results [47, 48].

The development of imaging diagnostics has been revolutionized by techniques such as PET and ultrasound with contrast media, as well as by the latest generation CT scanners which are able to detect tumor vascularization in a precise manner and thus evaluate the effectiveness of the response to treatment with anti-neoangiogenetic drugs.

The development of ultra specific tumor markers, by means of biotechnology, will enable a more precise identification of the tumor locations, and so the early identification of tumor and its staging so that treatment will be more effectively driven.

Genomics, which is able to build the "identity card" of tumors, will modify their classification which is currently based on pathologic anatomy, and so it will be able to vary the therapeutic indications, as well as anticipate the individual patient's response and the drug toxicity, so defining a tailored treatment of cancer.

However, it will be proteinomics that most influences future development: proteinomics is a large-scale analysis on the proteins expressed by the genome; its study is even more complicated than the study of the genome, because it involves the infinitely small and incredibly large numbers. Therefore, theoretically, it is more reliable because a genetic mutation may not express itself or, in contrast, it may express itself in a key protein of the cell replication; its study represents the *in vivo* reflection of molecular modifications. The aim is to obtain a proteinomic profile which however requires the use of complex computer systems capable of differentiating with 100% reliability between the different types of tumor. Furthermore, in case of tumors affecting the gastrointestinal tract, the extraction technique of these proteins may indicate different types of dysplasia from an initial adenoma and adenocarcinoma, and verify if the treatment has been complete or not. These techniques, while on the other hand so sophisticated, on the other are plagued with shortcomings due to a lack of homogeneity and validation with large patient populations.

The family forms of tumor (genetic predisposition) will be better comprehended, and so diagnosed in advance, and in theory it will be possible to identify the moment when a lesion can become precancerous and act at that moment. For the family forms, therefore, where the organ can present initial alterations on which the tumor evolves, prophylactic surgery will be developed; its timing will be guided by biology and, probably, prophylactic exeresis will become the basis of the new surgery.

In short, oncologic surgery can be rightfully defined "biosurgery", given the increasing frequency during the pre-, intra- and post-surgical phase of biological substances such as growth factors, cytokines, anti-adhesion molecules and neoangiogenesis inhibitors and biotechnologies which will allow the identification and targeting of evolving tumor formations not detectable by sight or palpation but rather by a surgical PET with marked FDG.

Future oncologic surgery will need to be of high quality and performed by a surgeon with some indispensable prerequisites: technical skills, specific education based on constantly evolving pathophysiologic experience, capability to standardize surgical methods and therapeutic protocols.

The oncologic surgeon will need to be a skilled surgeon, respecting the oncologic rules of tumor exeresis in relation to the organ involved and on the histological type of cancer, with an outstanding aptitude for collective decisions and an ability to cooperate effectively with pathologists, oncologists and radiotherapists. All of this is required in a well organized environment where advanced tumors will be no longer seen, only non-chemosensitive forms of a few centimeters in size.

References

1. Wiggers T, Jeekel J, Arends JW et al (1988) No-touch isolation tecnique in colon cancer: a controlled prospective trial. Br J Surg 75(5):409–415
2. Salsbury AJ (1975) The significance of the circulating cancer cell. Cancer Treat Rev 2(1):55–72
3. Sugarbaker PH, Corlew S (1982) Influence of surgical techniques on survival in patients with colorectal cancer. Dis Colon Rectum 25(6):545–557
4. Glaves D, Hubert RP, Weiss L (1988) Hematogenous dissemination of cells from human renal carcinomas. Br J Cancer 57: 32–35
5. Vlems FA, Ruers T J, Punt CJ et al (2003) Relevance of disseminated tumor in blood bone marrow of patients with solid epithelial tumors in perspective. EJSO 29:289–302
6. Klein CA, Blankestein TJ, Schmidr-Kittler O et al (2002) Genetic heterogenecity of single disseminated tumour cells in minimal residual cancer. Lancet 360:689–699
7. Fisher B, Fisher ER (1967) Barrier function of lymph node to tumor cells and erythrocytes. Cancer 20:1907–1913
8. Isono K, Sato H, Nakayama K (1991) Results of a nationwide study on the three-field lymph node dissection of esophageal cancer. Oncology 48(5):411–420
9. Hermanek P, Altendorf A (1981) Classification of colorectal carcinomas with regional lymphatic metastases. Pathol Res Pract 173(1–2):1–11
10. Hermanek P, Hutter RV, Sobin LH, Wagner G (1997) International Union Against Cancer. TNM atlas, IV edition. Springer, Berlin Heidelber New York
11. Hermanek P, Giegel P, Dworak O (1989) Two programs for examination of regional lymph nodes in colorectal carcinoma with regard to the new pN classification. Pathos Res Pract 185:867–872
12. Herrera L, Villareal JR (1992) Incidence of metastases from rectal adenocarcinoma in small lymph nodes detected by a clearing tecnique. Dis Colon Rectum 35(8):783–788
13. Morikawa E, Yasutomi M, Shindou K et al (1994) Distribution of metastatic lymph nodes in colorectal cancer by the modified clearing method. Dis Colon Rectum 37(3):219–223
14. Greenson JK, Isenhart CE, Rice R et al (1994) Identification of occult micrometastases in pericolic lymph nodes of Duke's B colorectal cancer patients using monoclonal antibodies against cytokeratin and CC49. Correlation with longterm survival. Cancer 73(3):563–569
15. Raj GV, Moreno JG, Gomella LG (1998) Utilization of polymerase chain reaction technology in the detection of solid tumors. Cancer 82:1419
16. Hayashi N, Ito I, Yanagisawa A et al (1995) Genetic diagnosis of lymph-node metastasis in colorectal cancer. Lancet 345(8960):1257–1259
17. Lindemann F, Schlimok G, Dirschell P (1992) Prognostic significance of micrometastatic tumor cells in bone marrow of colorectal cancer patients. Lancet 340(8821):685–689
18. Braun S, Pantel K, Muller P et al (2000) Cytokeratine-positive cells in bone marrow and sur-

vival of patients with stage I, II, or III breast cancer. N Engl J Med 342:525–533

19. Hosh SB, Braun S, Pantel K (2001) Characterization of disseminated tumor cells. Sem Surg Oncol 20:267–271

20. Hansen R, Wolf N, Knuechel R et al (1995) Tumor cells on blood shed from the surgical field. Arch Surg 130:387–393

21. Yamamoto K, Murae M, Yasuda M (1991) RGD - Containing peptides inhibit experimental peritoneal acceding of human ovarian cancer cells. Nippon Sanka Fujinka Gakkai Zasshi 43(12):1687–1692

22. Elias D, Gachot B, Bonvallot S et al (1997) Peritoneal carcinosis treated by complete excision and immediate postoperative intraperitoneal chemotherapy. Phase II study in 54 patients. Gastroenterol Clin Biol 21(3):181

23. Elias D, Cavalcanti A, Sabourin JC et al (1998) Results of 136 curative hepatectomies with a safety margin of less than 10mm for colorectal metastases. J Surg Oncol 69:88–93

24. Koo J, Fung K, Siu KF et al (1983) Recovery of malignant tumor cells from the right atrium duting hepatic resection for hepatocellular carcinoma. Surgery 52:1952–1956

25. Slade NS, Simmons RL, Yunis E (1975) Immunodepression after major surgery in normal patients. Surgery 78:363–372

26. Elias D, Farace F, Triebel F et al (1995) Phase I-II randomized study on pre-hepatectomy recombinant inerleukin-2 in patients with metastasis carcinoma of the colon and rectum. J Am Coll Surg 181:303–310

27. Baker DG, Masterson TM, Pacer R et al (1989) The influence of the surgical wound on local recurrence. Surgery 106:525–532

28. Elias D, Lasser P, Rougier P et al (1987) Early adjuvant intraportal chemotheraphy after curative hepatectomy for colorectal liver metastases. A pilot study. Eur J Surg Oncol 13:247–250

29. Romano F, Cesana G, Berselli M et al (2004) Biological histological, and clinical impact of preoperative IL-2 administration in radically operable gastric cancer patients. J Surg Oncol 88:240–247

30. Elias D (1992) La chirurgie dite de réduction tumorale: mythe ou realité? J Chir (Paris) 129:479–483

31. André T, Boni C, Mounedji-Boudiaf L et al (2004) Oxaliplatin, fluorouracil, and leucovorin as adjuvant treatment for colon cancer. N Engl J Med 350:2343–2351

32. Moertel CG, Fleming TH, Mac Donald JS et al (1990) Levamisole and fluorouracil for adjuvant therapy of resected carcinoma. N Engl J Surg 322:352–358

33. Elias D, Oueller JF (2001) Intraperitoneal chemohyperthermia. Rationale, technique, indication, and results. Surg Oncol Clin N Am 10:915–933

34. Verwaal VC, van Ruth S, de Bree E et al (2003) Randomized trial of cytoreduction and hypertermic intraperitoneal chemotherapy versus systemic chemotherapy and palliative surgery with peritoneal carcinomatosis from colorectal cancer. J Clin Oncol 21:3737–3743

35. Elias D, Sideris I, Pocard M et al (2004) Efficacy of intraperitoneal chemohypertermia with oxaliplatin in colorectal peritoneal carcinomatosis. Preliminary results in 24 patients. Ann Oncol 15:781–785

36. Adam R, Pascal G, Castaing D et al (2004) Tumor progression while on chemotherapy. A contraindication to liver resection for multiple colorectal metastases? Ann Surg 240:1052–1064

37. Peeters C, de Geus LF, Wetphal JR et al (2005) Decrease in circulating anti-angiogenic factor after removal of primary colorectal carcinoma coincides with increased metabolic activity of liver metastases. Surgery 137:246–249

38. Marie P, Cluner J (1910) Frequence des metastases viscérales chez les souri cancéreuses après ablation chirurgicale de leur tumeur. Bull Assoc Fr Etud Cancer 3:19–23

39. Buinauskas P, Mc Donald GO, Cole Wh (1958) Role of operative stress on the resistance of the experimental animal to inoculated cancer cells. Ann Surg 148:642–650

40. Murthy MS, Scanlon EF, Reid JK, Yang XF (1996) Pre, peri and postoperative chemotherapy for breast cancer: is one better than the other? J Surg Oncol 61:273–277

41. Elias D, Bonnay M, Puizzillou JM et al (2002) Heated intra-operative intraperitoneal oxaliplatin after complete resection of peritoneal carcinomatosis: pharmacokinetics and tissue distribution and tolerance. Ann Oncol 13:267–272
42. Elias D, Matsuhina T, Sideris L et al (2004) Heated intraoperative intraperitoneal oxaliplatin plus irinotecan after complete resection of peritoneal carcinomatosis: pharmacokinetics, tissue distribution and tolerance. Ann Oncol 15:1558–1565
43. Elias D, Liberale G, Vernerey D et al (2005) Hepatic and extrahepatic colorectal metastases: when resectable, their localization does not matter, but their total number has a prognostic impact. Ann Surg Oncol 12:900–909
44. Elias D, Youssef O, Sideris L et al (2004) Evolution of missing colorectal liver metastases following inductive chemotherapy and hepatectomy. J Surg Oncol 86:4–9
45. Weed DL, Greenwald P, Cullen JW (1990) The future of cancer prevention and control. Semin Oncol 17(4):504–509
46. Brown PD, Giavazzi R (1995) Matrix metalloproteinase inhibition: a review of anti-tumor activity. Ann Oncol 6 (10):967–974
47. Folkman J (1997) Angiogenesis and angiogenesis inhibition: an overview. EXS 79:1–8
48. O'Relly MS, Holmgren L, Chen C, Folkman J (1996) Angiostatin induces and sustains dormancy of human primary tumors in mice. Nat Med 2(6):689–692

Chapter 2

Cooperation between the Surgical Oncologist and the Pathologist

Antonio Bolognese, Francesco Borrini, Francesca Ricci, Paolo Meloni,
Federica Pulcini, Pietro L. Mingazzini

The diagnosis, treatment and follow up of oncologic patients require multidisciplinary working groups made up of a dedicated team of physicians. Over the last decade the multidisciplinary treatment of oncologic diseases has become increasingly integrated and decreasingly sequential. The aim of cooperation is to provide quality treatment and produce new knowledge through both basic and clinical research and medical education.

Cooperation in clinical practice leads to an individualized therapy and the selection of the most appropriate therapeutic approach, which is validated by protocols and therapeutic standards. Clearly, results depend on the efficiency and individual quality of the oncologic team, but adequate decisions are also determined by tumor stage and surgical removal. Therefore a key point is the interaction between the surgeon and the pathologist, as discussed below.

The pathologist has the opportunity of linking disease onset with the latter phases of disease progression, thus complementing the clinical data with pathological data in an evolutionary process.

As Ackerman wrote in a prior edition of "Surgical Pathology" [1]:

A good surgeon has not only technical dexterity (a fairly common commodity), but also, more importantly, good judgment and personal concern for his patient's welfare. The surgeon with a prepared mind and clear concept of the pathology of disease invariably is the one with good judgment. Without this background of knowledge, he will not recognize specific pathologic alterations at surgery nor will he have a clear concept of the limitations of his knowledge and therefore he will not know when to call the pathologist to help him. Without this basic knowledge, he may improve his technical ability but never his judgment. One might say that with him his ignorance is refined rather than his knowledge broadened.

We can analyze the cooperation between the surgical oncologist and the pathologist by answering the following two questions: "What can surgical oncologist do for the pathologist?" and "What can pathologist do for the surgical oncologist?"

A. Bolognese, L. Izzo (eds.), *Surgery in Multimodal Management of Solid Tumors.*
©Springer-Verlag Italia 2009

What Can the Surgical Oncologist Do for the Pathologist?

A histopathological report is an important medical document (and unfortunately also a medico-legal document). It includes any relevant macroscopic and microscopic features of the tumor, and provides an interpretation of them for the clinician.

It can be difficult, or even impossible, for the pathologist to produce an accurate and complete report in the absence of appropriate clinical information or a large enough sample from the surgeon. For an optimal report the pathologist needs to know the patient's age, sex, past and present personal and family clinical history, as well as information regarding imaging, previous surgery, chemotherapy or other therapies done prior to surgery. An appropriate pathological examination form should be written in clear and legible writing and include the patient's name, surname, date of birth, sex, clinical history, surgical treatment and any information relevant to the surgical oncologist. Any material, either in fixative media or fresh, should be entirely sent to the pathologist. Lesions to be examined need to be completely excised, with a normal tissue rim.

When this kind of surgery is too invasive the surgical oncologist can choose from a number of different procedures, such as incision biopsy, punch biopsy, shave biopsy, core biopsy, fine needle biopsy or fine needle aspiration cytology. Although the latter three techniques are appropriate for superficial lesions, in the presence of lymph node masses or visceral neoplasms, sampling can be inadequate even under ultrasound guidance. Biopsy information tends to be limited, since only part of the lesion is under study.

The identification and orientation of the correct biopsy technique is fundamental for an accurate diagnosis, so in difficult cases the surgical oncologist must cooperate with the pathologist to identify the lesion position, anatomical boundaries and surgical margins. The surgical oncologist can also mark the interested areas, (e.g. the resection of a sarcoma) when this is near the periosteal margin, the surgeon can stitch the nearest point. Otherwise, when performing the sentinel node procedure, marking the afferent lymphatic dye entry can be useful to precisely examine the most common micrometastasis location.

Although a diagnosis can be made easily with limited clinical data, clear and effective communication between the pathologist and the surgical oncologist is clearly necessary to avoid inadequate treatment, which can damage patient outcome and clinical practice.

What Can the Pathologist Do for the Surgical Oncologist?

Often the surgical oncologist knows the diagnosis before surgery is performed, but is less informed with regard to tumor spread, invasion of adjacent sites, positive margins, nerve infiltration, lymph nodes or metastasis to other organs. Therefore, the surgical oncologist needs any available information to appropriately plan surgical treatment and adjuvant therapies.

The surgical procedure is made up of three distinct phases: before, during and after surgery. In the preoperative phase the surgeon needs to determine the histological type and grading of the neoplasm in order to establish an accurate and multidisciplinary tumor approach. During surgery rapid and precise interaction between the surgeon and the pathologist guarantee adequate treatment depending on specific guidelines and individual case data, which are unknown prior to surgery. During the third phase the drawing up of the pathological report expresses the surgeon's work (gross), the pathologist's knowledge and assessment (microscopy) and conclusions, and is completed with additional data such as immunohistochemistry and molecular biology (diagnosis).

When writing up the report the pathologist must ask himself what information the surgical oncologist needs to get out of it. Cooperation between the pathologist, surgeon and oncologist can be the basis for a useful and necessary schematic report, such as the Sidney Melanoma Unit Synoptic Report [2]. Not all cases, however, can be outlined in this way, in part due to surgical complexity, in part to the pathologist's particular inclination.

Any uncertainty with regard to lesion progression must be included in the report, with the suggestion of seeking a more expert second opinion, so as to avoid any unnecessary aggressive surgical treatment.

What We Do at Our Institute

At our Institute we always seek to cooperate to satisfy any pathologic and surgical demands at the sickbed. Generally we communicate extensively before, during and after the surgical procedure, especially in cases when the benign or malignant nature of a mass is not clear. We believe in the need to always remember our limits, and that the burden of our diagnosis, whether brilliant or mistaken, does not lie heavily on us alone.

To clarify our behavior in oncologic matters, we shall present two tumors which are frequently treated at our Institute: colorectal carcinoma and mammary carcinoma.

Colorectal Carcinoma

The gross examination of the colon cancer specimen, together with knowledge of the anatomy and its variants, are vital. The size and width of the mesorectum differ from patient to patient. Some patients have a small mesorectum and thus have a greater risk of radial margin infiltration even for small tumors, whereas others with an ample mesorectum have a clean radial margin in spite of widespread tumors [3]. After receiving the specimen, the pathologist must locate the anterior and posterior portions, the surgically created surfaces, and closely watch for lacerations and perforations. After opening the bowel and carefully avoiding the tumor, the pathologist inks the area and puts in fixative for 24–48 h.

The surgery quality evaluation in mesorectum resection is made grossly, by examining the distance between the tumor and the inked resection margin, and microscopically, by marking the distance between the marked margin and the nearest neoplastic cell.

We consider an excision incomplete when tumor cells are less than 1 mm from the stained margin. The modes of involvement, whether direct, discontinuous, venous or neural, all confer a poor prognosis [4]. As well as the radial margin, the distal margin needs to be considered, especially in rectal resection, because the frequency of distal involvement is around 1–2% in different studies [5]. With regard to oncologic surgery in general, and not only in colorectal cancer, an accurate lymph node count is a key point [6]. Lymph-node sampling and the metastatic lymph-node ratio, as shown by several authors, are fundamental parameters for evaluating hospital performance, for allowing an evidence-based management plan to be made for the patient and for accurately indicating prognosis [7]. We do not use any particular technique for the visualization of lymph nodes, but rather follow the indications proposed by Ratto [8] and Potter [9]: a good lymph-node count is possible without fat-clearance, by adequate mesenteric tissue fixation and a meticulous search. Fat clearance methods are too expensive and problematic for routine use [10]. In addition, we have recently been defining the sentinel node procedure, according to the Gustav-Roussy experience, to improve staging for N0 patients [11]. In our procedure we inject the blue dye ex vivo after the excision, and then we dissect the marked lymph node directly for a separate examination (Figs, 2.1 and 2.2). When <0.5 mm the lymph node is completely paraffin embedded, and when >0.5 mm we place it in two cassettes. We cut multiple sections from every lymph node, some of which are then colored in hematoxylin-eosin. If no metastasis is evident in the slides, we use anti-cytokeratin AE1/AE2 staining.

Close cooperation is also present for rectal cancer patients after neoadjuvant treatment. After surgery the specimen is sent directly to the Surgical Pathology Unit where it is opened with the surgeon's assistance, and the tumor site is identified. After 24–48 h the whole tumor site is sampled. With a standard hematoxylin-eosin staining, we examine the suspicious area. If there is still no tumor we proceed with AE1/AE2 anti-cytokeratin staining to apply the TRG (tumor regression grade), according to Dworak [12] (Table 2.1).

In conclusion in metastatic colorectal carcinoma we analyze the expression of epithelial growth-factor receptor (EGFR). EGFR is highly expressed in 25–77% of colorectal carcinomas, and is associated with poor prognosis [14] and radio resistance, although EGFR-positive patients can undergo cetuximab treatment.

Mammary Carcinoma

With regard to mammary carcinoma, the surgical sample has to be sent immediately to the laboratory, since only the pathologist can make the sampling.

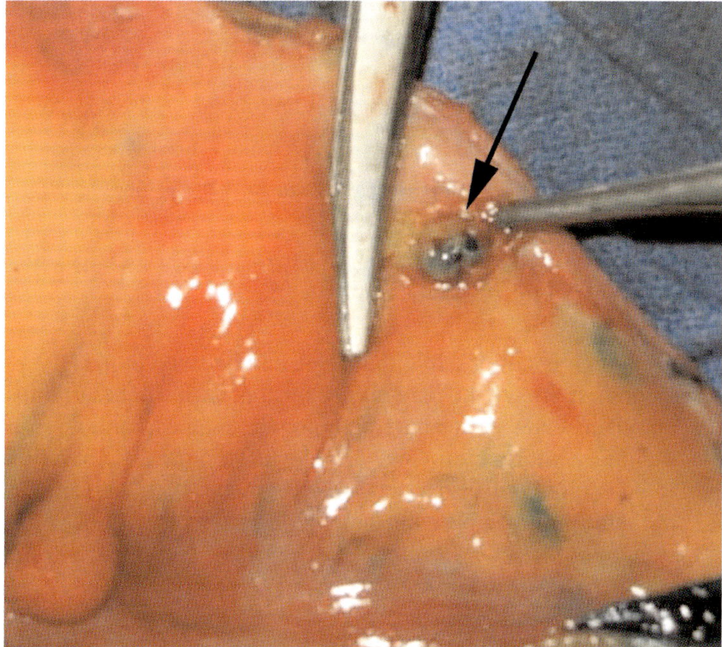

Fig. 2.1 Colorectal cancer: sentinel node (*arrow*) after ex-vivo inoculation of toluidine blue dye (kindly granted by Prof. P Lasser, Institut Gustave Roussy, Villejuif, France)

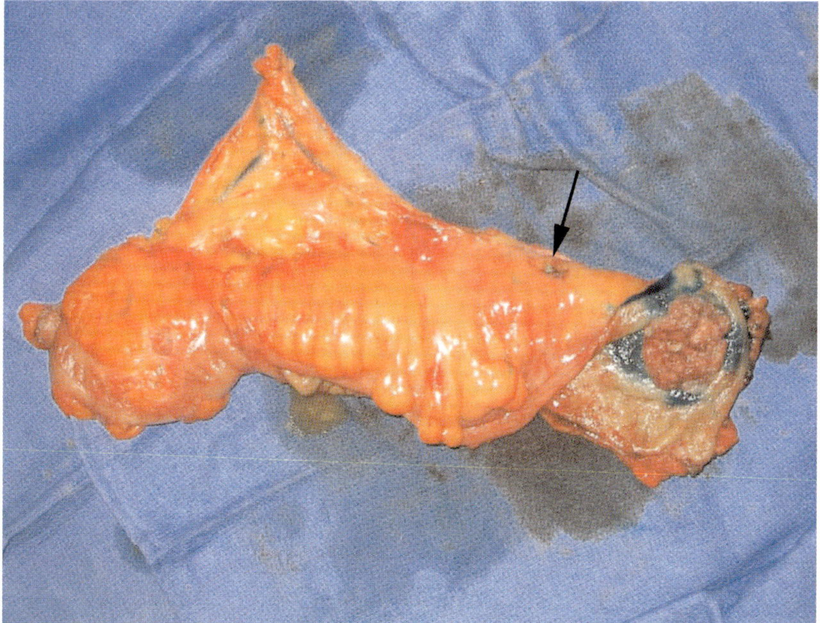

Fig. 2.2 Colorectal cancer: sentinel node (*arrow*)

Table 2.1 Tumor regression grade (TRG) according to Dworak et al., cited in [13]

Grade 0	No regression
Grade 1	Dominant tumor mass with obvious fibrosis and/or vasculopathy
Grade 2	Dominantly fibrotic changes with few tumor cells or groups (easy to find)
Grade 3	Very few(difficult microscopically) tumor cells in fibrotic tissue with or without mucous substance
Grade 4	No tumor cells, only a fibrotic mass (total regression or response)

Obviously when this is not possible the tissue can be fixed in pH7 10% formalin. The surgeon first orients the mammary excision, with stitches or clips for X-ray study, and then sends an accurate pathological request, with an orientation scheme and clinical information (Fig. 2.3). When lesions are not palpable the surgeon also adds radiological data and images for an accurate sampling (Fig. 2.4). The first question to answer for the pathologist, in the era of conservative surgical treatment, is the accuracy of the excision [15]. Margins are evaluated on two occasions: first during surgery with a predominantly gross examination, when we evaluate the minimal distance from the tumor, and second at light microscopy examination, when we evaluate the distance between the inked margin and the nearest tumor cells. We thoroughly excise the nodule, when small in toto, and we also take blocks of the entire suspicious area.

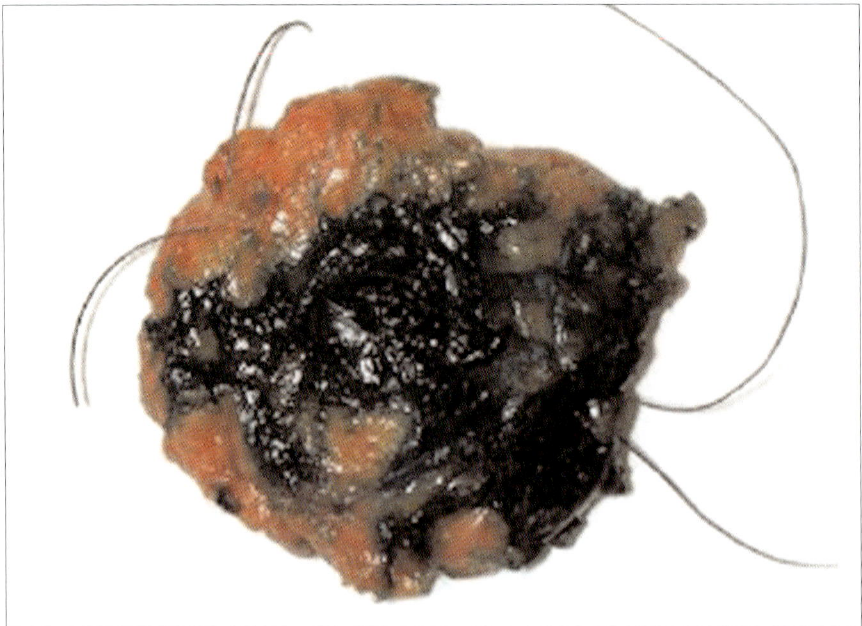

Fig. 2.3 Quadrantectomy

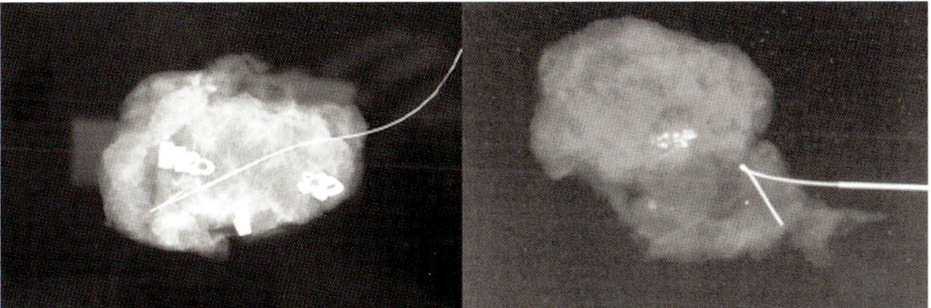

Fig. 2.4 Mammography

All the lesions are defined by histotype, differentiation, in situ component, cutaneous, neural or vascular invasion. Moreover we study the molecular profiling of the tumor, and evaluate estrogen and progesterone receptors, proliferation index, and HER2/neu overexpression, which reflects HER2 amplification which despite being correlated with a poor prognosis, HER2-positive patients can be treated with Herceptin [16]. In oncology, as stated above, the lymph-node study is fundamental, and in selected cases we apply the sentinel node procedure in the search for micrometastasis and isolated tumor cells by immunohistochemistry (Fig. 2.5). In other cases we look for a high lymph-node count. Also in breast pathology, with a multidisciplinary approach, we meticulously study the post neoadjuvant specimens, also with the use of immunohistochemistry when needed, to evaluate the treatment response according to Miller [17] (Table 2.2).

In addition to our daily efforts at achieving excellent care for cancer patients, at our Institute we always seek to cooperate in research projects to improve patient management. Our studies have been based on archive blocks, sometimes on fresh tissue, with significant involvement of the surgeon-pathologist alliance to obtain representative samples without reducing subsequent diagnostic accuracy.

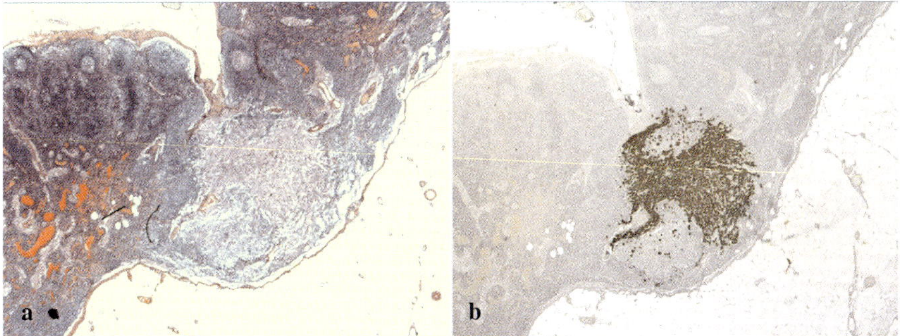

Fig. 2.5 Mammary ductal carcinoma: lymph node micrometastasis. **a** H&E. **b** Immunohistochemistry CK

Table 2.2 Neoadjuvant therapy response histopathologic grading according to Miller et al., cited in [18]

Primary site of response

Grade 1	Some alteration to individual malignant cells but no reduction in overall numbers as compared with the pre-treatment core biopsy
Grade 2	A minor loss of invasive tumor cells but overall cellularity still high
Grade 3	A moderate reduction in tumor cells up to an estimated 90% loss
Grade 4	A marked disappearance of invasive tumor cells such that only small clusters of widely dispersed cells could be detected
Grade 5	No invasive tumor, i.e. only in situ disease or stoma tumor remained

Axillary LN response (proposed)

N-A	True axillary LN negative
N-B	Axillary LN positive and no therapeutic effects
N-C	Axillary LN positive but evidence of partial pathologic response
N-D	Initially axillary LN positive but converted to LN negative after PST

Currently we are working on a new project about bone marrow minimal residual disease (MRD) in colorectal and mammary carcinomas which involves surgeons, pathologists, molecular biologists and oncologists. The aim of the study is to demonstrate that apart from being a prognostic factor, MRD can be used for treatment monitoring and specifically targeted therapy [19]. The persistence of MRD after treatment suggests further adjuvant treatment [20].

This kind of close cooperation is necessary now more than ever, since in the future we hope to achieve the early diagnosis of tumors before invasion and metastasis, as well as improve staging and classification systems, evaluate tumor aggressiveness and predict treatment response [21].

Lastly, with regard to medical training, the presence of pathology residents and surgery residents in our daily practice leads to a close interaction early in their training, which is essential for their future cooperation.

References

1. Rosai J (2004) Rosai and Ackerman's Surgical Pathology. 9th ed, vol 1, Mosby, St Louis, pp 1–6
2. Thompson JF, Scolyer RA (2004) Cooperation between surgical oncologist and pathologist: a key element of multidisciplinary care for patient with cancer. Pathology 36(5):496–503
3. Qiurke P, Morris E (2007) Reporting colorectal cancer. Histopathology 50:103–112
4. Birbeck KF, Macklin CP, Tiffin NJ et al (2002) Rates of circunferential resection margin involvement vary between surgeons and predict outcomes in rectal cancer. Ann Surg 235:449–457
5. Guillou PJ, Quirke P, Bosanquet N et al (2003) The MRC CLASSIC trial: result of short-term endpoints. Br J Cancer 88:S21

6. Bolognese A, Barbarosos A, Borrini F et al (2001) Standardizzazione delle attuali metodiche chirurgiche ed anatomopatologiche per la rilevazione linfonodale e significato prognostico delle micrometastasi. Archivio ed Atti della Società Italiana di Chirurgia,Volume 2, Roma, pp 11–24

7. Bilchik AJ, Compton C (2007) Close collaboration between surgeon and pathologist is essential for accurate staging of early colon cancer. Ann Surg 245(6):864–866

8. Ratto C, Sofo L, Ippoliti M et al (1999) Accurate lymph-node detection in colorectal specimens resected for cancer is of prognostic significance. Dis Colon Rectum 42(2):143–154 discussion 154–158

9. Poller DN (2000) Method of specimen fixation and pathological dissection ofcolorectal cancer influences retrieval of lymph nodes and tumour nodal stage. Eur J Surg Oncol 26(8):758–762

10. Noda N, Sasako M, Yamaguchi N et al (1998) Ignoring small lymph nodes can be a mejor cause of staging error in gastric cancer. Br J Surg 85:831–34

11. Liberale G, Lasser P, Sabourin JC et al (2007) Sentinel lymph nodes of colorectal carcinoma: reappraisal of 123 cases. Gastroenterol Clin Biol 31:281–285

12. Dworak O, Keilholz L, Hoffman A et al (1997) Pathological features of rectal cancer after preoperative radiochemotherapy. Int J Colorect Dis 12:19–23

13. Benzoni E, Intersimone D, Terrosu G et al (2006) Prognostic value of tumour regression grading and depth of neoplastic infiltration within the perirectal fat after combined neoadiuvant chemo-radiotherapy and surgery for rectal cancer. J Clin Pathol 59b:505–512

14. Kopp R, Rothbauer E, Ruge M (2003) Clinical implications of the EGF receptor/ligand system for tumor progression and survival in gastrointestinal carcinomas: evidence for new therapeutic options. Recent Results. Cancer Res 162:115–132. Review Dis Col Rectum 46:1931–1939

15. FONCaM (2003) I tumori della mammella, linee guida sulla diagnosi, il trattamento e la riabilitazione. Società Italiana di Senologia, Scientific Press, Milan

16. Slamon DJ, Leyland-Jones B, Shak S et al (2001) Use of chemotherapy plus monoclonal antibody against HER2 for metastatic breast cancer that overexpressed HER2. N Engl J Med 344(17):783–792

17. Smith IC, Miller ID (2001) Issue involvement in research into neoadjuvant treament for breast cancer. Anticancer Drugs 12(Suppl 1):S25-S29

18. Kuroi K, Toi M, Tsuda H et al (2006) Issue in the assessment of pathologic effect of primary systemic therapy for breast cancer. Breast Cancer 13:38–48

19. Bolognese A, Barbarosos A,Biacchi D et al (2002) Basi fisiopatologiche e ruolo della chirurgia oncologica nella formazione del chirurgo generale. Ann Ital Chir LXXIII 6:553–561

20. Janni W, Rack B, Lindemann K et al (2005) Detection of micrometastatic disease in bone marrow: is it ready for prime time? Oncologist 10:480–492

21. Marian Grade, Beker H, Ghadimi BM et al (2004) The impact of molecular pathology in oncology: the clinician's perspective. Cell Oncol 26:275–278

Chapter 3

Molecular Biology and Genetics of Cancer

Alberto Gulino

Introduction

The concept that cancer is a multi-step process caused by genetically- and epigenetically-determined abnormal gene function is now well established. Gain-of-function or loss-of-function changes affect a number of genes that control cellular processes such as cell cycle, apoptosis and differentiation and that consequently behave as oncogenes or tumor suppressors, respectively. It is also well established that several genetic hits are required to trigger cell transformation and malignant progression of cancer, in which the altered functions of each oncogene or tumor suppressor contribute, in a coordinated way, to compose the complex network of the cancer phenotypic traits [1, 2]. Elucidating how such gene function diversity is generated during the tumorigenic events is an unanswered question. Although tremendous advances in knowledge have occurred in recent years, there is still no clear understanding in this field.

Genetic and Epigenetic Basis of Cancer: Oncogenes and Tumor Suppressor Genes

Genetic Mutations

A mechanism of gene function change is provided by the occurrence of DNA mutations which accumulate in the cell because of its genomic instability. Genomic instability is caused by ineffective DNA repair systems which are unable to overcome genotoxic stresses. A number of major enzymatic systems are involved in the repair of damaged DNA (e.g. double strand DNA break, DSB [Nbs1/MRE1/RAD50 complex] and mismatch repair, MMR [MLH1, MSH2, MSH6, PMS, PMS2]). Mutations in DSB and MMR genes characterize a number of human diseases that are associated with a predisposition to cancer. For instance, the Ataxia-Telangiectasia and the Nijmegen diseases are autosomal recessive disorders due to mutations of the ATM and NBS1 genes, respectively, and predispose to lymphoproliferative disorders. A subset of colorectal cancers

A. Bolognese, L. Izzo (eds.), *Surgery in Multimodal Management of Solid Tumors.*
©Springer-Verlag Italia 2009

also display mutations of MMR genes whose defective function causes the accumulation of mutations of mononucleotide repeats in cancer-related genes (TGFbetaRII, Bax, IGFIIR), thus contributing to carcinogenesis. Interestingly, multiple defects of DNA repair genes can coexist in cancer cells, thus amplifying the genomic instability. Indeed, we observed that the poly(T)11 repeat within human MRE11 intron 4 is mutated in MMR-deficient colorectal cancer, leading to aberrant splicing and truncated defective protein [3].

A low percentage of breast and ovarian carcinomas (approximately 5–10%) are caused by a genetic susceptibility and some of them are related to genetic mutations in BRCA1 and BRCA2 genes. Genetic testing of individuals belonging to high-risk families, likely to harbor a germline mutation in a BRCA gene, is currently employed to address the clinical management of mutation carriers [4 and reviewed in 5].

Epigenetic Control of Gene Function

In addition to genetic mutations, epigenetic misregulation of gene expression is a critical feature of cancer. Methylation status of CpG islands in gene promoters is crucial for controlling gene expression. For instance, a number of tumor suppressor genes are silenced through hypermethylation. An appropriate histone acetylation status is also a critical event for the control of gene transcription and results from a balance of acetyltransferase (HAT) and histone deacetylase (HDAC) enzymatic activities. HDAC have been related to the pathogenesis of cancer and small-molecule HDAC inhibitors are employed in clinical trials as effective antitumor drugs [reviewed in 6].

Alternative Splicing Unveils Oncogene Function

Finally, alternative splicing is emerging as a mechanism for the tuning of gene function and, if misregulated, as a critical event responsible for tumorigenesis. Indeed, diverse proteins may arise from a single transcript through alternative splicing. We have recently described how a misregulated alternative splicing can generate aberrant proteins provided with oncogenic properties. The first example is a novel oncogene (TrkAIII) identified in neuroblastoma, a highly aggressive malignant childhood tumor of neural crest origin [7].

Neurotrophin tyrosine kinase receptor type 1 (TrkA), a member of the tyrosine kinase neurotrophin receptor family that includes TrkB and TrkC, is the preferred receptor for nerve growth factor (NGF) and is critical for the development and maturation of central and peripheral nervous systems, regulating proliferation, differentiation and apoptosis. We identified a novel alternative TrkA splice variant, TrkAIII, with deletion of exons 6, 7, and 9 and functional extracellular IG-C1 and N-glycosylation domains, which is preferentially expressed in undifferentiated early neural progenitors, human neuroblastomas and a subset of other neural crest-derived tumors. This NGF-unresponsive isoform is oncogenic and promotes tumorigenic neuroblastoma cell behavior resulting from spontaneous tyrosine kinase activity and phosphatidylinositol 3-kinase (PI3K)/Akt/NF-kB but not Ras/MAPK signaling. TrkAIII antagonizes NGF/TrkAI signaling, which is responsible for neuroblastoma growth arrest and differentiation through Ras/MAPK. This provides a mechanism for converting NGF/TrkA/Ras/MAPK antioncogenic signals to TrkAIII/PI3K/Akt/NF-kB tumor-promoting signals during tumor progression of neuroblastoma [7].

In another neural tumor, medulloblastoma, we have identified an alternatively spliced ErbB4 receptor isoform that sustains tumorigenesis. A subset of medulloblastomas displays levels of the ErbB-4-CYT-1 over the CYT-2 isoforms generated by alternative splicing of the cytoplasmic domain. CYT-1 includes a PI3K-binding site, that is missing in CYT-2, thus enhancing the resistance to apoptosis by activation of PI3K/Akt and highlighting the oncogenic function of this alternatively spliced isoform [8].

A similar alternative splicing has been reported to contribute to the pathogenesis of T cell acute lymphoblastic leukemia (T-ALL). We have described that Notch3 signaling, which is hyperactive in human T-ALL, enhances the expression of the RNA binding protein HuD which in turn promotes alternative splicing of Ikaros transcription factors, generating dominant negative isoforms which sustain leukemogenesis [9].

MicroRNAs: A Novel Class of Genes Involved in Cancer

In addition to protein-encoding genes, a second class of genes producing small noncoding RNAs (i.e. microRNAs) has been discovered over the last few years. These RNAs are short molecules (18- to 24-nucleotides) that bind to cis-regulatory elements mainly present in the 3' UTR of mRNAs, resulting in translational inhibition or mRNA degradation. Mature microRNAs are generated from longer precursors through sequential processing by two members of the RNase III enzyme family, Drosha (pri-microRNA) and subsequently Dicer (pre-microRNA). MicroRNAs have emerged as important regulatory factors involved in developmental processes, such as neural progenitor cell growth and differentiation. The critical role played by microRNAs is also suggested by their altered expression observed in a large number of malignancies [10]. In addition, the ability of some miRNAs to target oncogenes or oncosuppressors indicates their role in tumorigenesis [10].

Although microRNAs play a crucial role in neuronal development, so far specific changes in their expression patterns have been described only in neural crest derived neuroblastoma [11]. Indeed, we have recently identified a crucial role for three neuronal microRNAs (miR-9, miR-125a and miR-125b) in controlling human neuroblastoma growth via the repression of a common target, the truncated isoform of the neurotrophin receptor Trk-C, which is able to promote cell proliferation. Truncated Trk-C receptor is generated from alternative splicing of *TrkC* mRNA, resulting in a receptor deleted of tyrosine kinase domain. Therefore, by targeting only the alternatively spliced TrkC, these microRNAs unbalance the full length protein over the truncated TrkC. Consistently with their function, these microRNAs were found to be down-modulated in primary neuroblastoma tumors [11].

Targeting Oncogenes and Tumor Suppressors: Gene Therapy

Accumulation of genetic and epigenetic alteration is a hallmark of cancer. Therefore, cancer gene therapy (i.e. introducing genetic material into cells) represents an ideal treatment strategy for targeting these underlying molecular abnormalities and restoring cell functions. Cancer gene therapy can also be combined with other treatment modalities (e.g. radiotherapy and chemotherapy) to enhance radiosensitivity or cytotoxicity in tumor compared to normal tissues. In addition to targeting specific genes underlying deregulated cell functions (e.g. angiogenesis, silencing abnormal cellular pathways, subverted survival, immune escape), cytotoxic approaches such as virus directed enzyme prodrug therapy or oncolytic viral therapy are currently used and investigated. Although they are a promising therapeutic approach, nevertheless very few clinical trials reach phase III, underscoring a lack of significant clinical advancement facing such a huge challenging task. Indeed, the most critical issues in cancer gene therapy are (a) the choice of the modalities of gene transfer (e.g. viral vector such as retroviruses, adenoviruses, adeno-associated viruses, lentiviruses, poxviruses, herpes viruses), (b) the targeting strategies by which only a sufficient number of tumor cell are reached and (c) avoiding the associated risks (e.g. insertional mutagenesis, transfer into reproductive cells, immune response).

Cancer Stem Cells and Relationships between Aberrant Cell Development and Tumorigenesis: The Paradigm of Brain Tumors

It is becoming increasingly clear that cancer may be considered as an aberrant morphogenetic process in which molecular signaling pathways regulating cell development are subverted. The link between the biology of cancer and developmental biology is underscored not only by the processes controlling tissue pattern formation during embryogenesis, but also by the mechanisms regulating tissue pattern maintenance such as post-embryonic tissue renewal and repair in response to injury. Indeed, morphogenetic embryonic development and post-embryonic tissue pattern maintenance are sustained by stem cells undergoing proliferation and differentiation events delineating sequential steps of cell lineage commitment throughout cell progenitor transitions until a fully differentiated phenotype. Stem cells are characterized by the ability to give rise to daughter cells with equal developmental potential and unlimited replication (i.e. self-renewal) and also capable of generating more restricted differentiated cell types (i.e. pluripotency).

The first link between the biology of development and the biology of cancer is given by the discovery that stem cells with similar properties have also been identified in most cancers (cancer stem cells or tumor initiating cells), suggesting that tumors arise and grow as a result of the formation of cancer stem cells, which may constitute a never ending reservoir for tumor maintenance and progression. Therefore, stem cells have been suggested as candidate "cell of origin" of cancer. Since stem cells are relatively long-lived and may go through various replicative cycles, they may have more opportunity to accumulate the multiple additional mutations required to increase the proliferation rate, thus producing a manifest cancer.

Further evidence of the relationship between aberrant morphogenetic process and cancer is given by the fact that tissue pattern embryonic formation or post-embryonic maintenance share with malignant transformation a number of regulatory signaling pathways (e.g. Hedgehog, Notch, Wnt) which undergo a specific misregulation in cancer. Therefore, a deeper understanding beyond the boundaries of cancer biology and developmental biology, addressing the investigation of the mechanisms that control normal development, is likely to provide insight into the molecular basis of cancer.

Medulloblastoma: A Paradigm of Brain Tumorigenesis Caused by Subverted Development

Paradigmatic evidence of the subversion of cell progenitor development as a cause of malignant transformation is provided by medulloblastoma, the most common (3.3 in 100,000 children) childhood brain malignancy. Current treatment approaches (a combination of surgery, chemotherapy and radiotherapy), although improving survival (56% 5-year survival), still have only limited efficacy and, most importantly, severe long-term side effects. Novel therapeutic strategies are thus needed based on specific molecular targets controlling crucial events of the cancer cell biology. Among the various signaling pathways that are misregulated in medulloblastoma, Hedgehog plays a crucial pathogenic role.

Hedgehog is one of the most potent morphogens involved in both invertebrate and vertebrate development. It was first discovered in *Drosophila* as a regulator of segment polarity in the embryo [12]. Since then, accumulating evidence has shown that Hedgehog is a master regulator of mammalian stem/progenitor cell behavior in physiologic and neoplastic contexts. Hedgehog signaling pathway activation is triggered by the interaction of Hedgehog ligands (i.e. Shh, Ihh and Dhh) with the inhibitory transmembrane receptor Patched (Ptc), thus relieving its inhibitory activity upon Smoothened (Smo) which in turn activates the downstream transcription factors belonging to the Gli family (Gli1, Gli2 and Gli3) [reviewed in 12].

Medulloblastoma is believed to arise from oncogenic transformation of the cerebellar granule cell progenitors (GCPs). The physiological control of GCP development is sustained by Purkinje cell-produced Shh which keeps GCPs proliferating and undifferentiated in the outer region of the External Germinal Layer (EGL). Interruption of Hedgehog signaling allows GCPs to exit cell cycle and to start a differentiation program in the inner region of the EGL. The first evidence that subversion of Hedgehog signaling is responsible for the onset of medulloblastoma is provided by the tumor formation observed in Ptc1$^{+/-}$ mice and subsequently in transgenics expressing *Smo* carrying a constitutive activatory mutation, indicating that withdrawal of the Hedgehog activity prevents tumorigenesis. Indeed, maintenance of activated Hedgehog signaling leads to GCP overgrowth and eventually to malignant transformation. Loss- or gain-of-function mutations of *Ptch1* or *Smo*, respectively, have also been reported in about 25% of human medulloblastomas [reviewed in 13]: however, the Hedgehog pathway appears to be hyperactive in a larger number of medulloblastomas. These observations suggest the presence additional genetic or epigenetic hits in pathways which in some way control Hedgehog signaling. In this regard a group of tumors which clustered with concurrent deletion of chromosome 17p also displayed high Hedgehog signaling signature in the absence of known mutations of components of the Hedgehog pathway [14].

A role for the loss of an additional negative regulator of Hedgehog signaling in medulloblastoma is also suggested by our previous observations describing the identification of the *REN*^{KCTD11} gene. Disruption of the *REN* gene represents a link between unrestrained Hedgehog signaling and chromosome 17p deletion in medulloblastoma. This latter genetic alteration is most frequently observed in medulloblastoma (up to 50%) and is believed to underlie the loss of one or more putative tumor suppressors [13]. We have suggested that *REN* is a novel putative tumor suppressor which is upregulated by EGF, retinoic acid and NGF and is expressed early during embryonic development, first in neural fold epithelium during gastrulation and, subsequently, throughout the neural tube and in postmitotic neuroblasts of the ventricular encephalic epithelium [15]. In the developing cerebellum, *REN* is expressed to a higher extent in non proliferating cells of the inner EGL and in IGL differentiated granule neurons rather than in high proliferating outer EGL GCPs, that instead express Gli1, a sensitive readout of active Hedgehog signaling [16]. The pattern of REN expression is consistent with a role in the control of the differentiation and growth of GCPs. Indeed, REN promotes growth arrest, neuronal differentiation and apoptosis of cultured GCPs [16]. Interestingly, the effects of REN appear to be due to the antagonism on the Hedgehog pathway, as indicated by its ability to inhibit Gli-dependent transcriptional activation of target genes as well as the Shh-induced mitogenic activity and the Shh-suppressed neuronal differentiation of cultured GCPs [16]. Conversely, inactivation of REN function in cultured GCPs resulted in both enhancement of Hedgehog signaling and increased cell proliferation together with reduced neuronal differentiation [16]. These observations suggest a role for REN as an inhibitory signal required for withdrawing GCP expansion at the outer to inner EGL transition, in an early phase of development.

Interestingly, human *REN* maps to 17p13.2 and is both deleted and silenced in a methylation-dependent way in a consistent number (40%) of medulloblastomas [17]. Restoring high *REN* expression inhibits medulloblastoma growth by negatively regulating Gli function [17]. Therefore, the loss of such an inhibitory signal, as a consequence of 17p deletion, may lead to the uncontrolled GCP overgrowth linked to medulloblastoma development.

Hedgehog Pathway, Stem Cells and Cancer Stem Cells

Hedgehog signaling has been described to play a critical role in brain morphogenesis, by regulating the ventral patterning of the neural tube as well as the proliferation of precursor cells in the dorsal brain [12]. To this regard, a specific essential function for Hedgehog signaling has also been described in the maintenance and self-renewal of neural progenitors in stem-cell niches located in several regions of the embryonic, post-natal, and adult brain. For instance, in the developing embryonic cortex, Hedgehog signaling regulates the number and growth of cells with stem cell properties and maintains stem cell niches in which these cells exist and proliferate. Similar observations have been reported in the post-natal forebrain subventricular zone, the stem cell niche of adult mammalian brain [18].

Brain tumors (including medulloblastoma) have been described to contain cancer stem cells [19], representing both the potential cell of origin of the tumor and a reservoir responsible for disease recurrence. Indeed, cancer stem cells appear to be resistant to conventional cytotoxic treatments. This is a major challenge for cancer control, thus needing more targeting therapeutic strategies able to affect their stemness identity. To this end, the Hedgehog pathway is a good candidate as a therapeutic target: indeed, it is involved in the pathogenesis of a large number of tumors in addition to medulloblastoma (glioblastoma, basal cell skin cancer, rhabdomyosarcoma, prostate, breast, pancreas and upper gastrointestinal tract, lung, melanoma) where it is emerging to sustain cancer stem cell population (e.g glioblastoma).

We have recently identified a tumor suppressor role for Numb in regulating the Hedgehog/Gli1 function in cerebellar progenitors and medulloblastoma cells [20], thus providing novel insights into the link between ubiquitination-based Gli processing and neural stem/progenitor cell development and thereby derived tumors. Indeed, Numb is a major determinant of asymmetric cell division by which daughter cells acquire binary cell fates including self-renewal versus differentiation ability. Such a role has been described in *Drosophila* larval brain neuroblasts which divide asymmetrically to generate either self-renewing neuroblasts or terminally differentiating ganglion mother cell (GMC) daughters. Numb asymmetrically distributes into the GMC to inhibit cell self-renewal. Interestingly, when the machinery that regulates asymmetric cell divisions is disrupted (e.g. loss of function mutants of *Drosophila* Numb or Aurora-A) these neuroblasts begin dividing symmetrically and become tumorigenic. These observations underscore a function for Numb in limiting stemness in *Drosophila* neuroblasts, likely due to impairment of asymmetric cell division and self-renewal of progenitor cells [21].

A similar asymmetric distribution and function in neural progenitor cells has also been described in mammalian cells. In keeping with its ability to promote neuronal differentiation, Numb deficiency in mouse cerebellum prevents the differentiation of GCP which accumulate in the EGL [22]. Accordingly, we have described downregulated expression of Numb in the outer layer of EGL where proliferating progenitor cells reside [20]. In contrast Numb expression is observed in inner EGL and internal granule layer where granule cell progenitors stop proliferating and differentiate [20]. Interestingly we have identified a previously unsuspected role of this protein as a negative regulator of Hedgehog signaling via triggering ubiquitin-dependent degradation of Gli1 [20].

Post-synthetic protein modifications by ubiquitin-dependent processes have emerged as crucial mechanisms by which protein function is controlled. Ubiquitin can be covalently linked to lysine residues of target proteins as polyubiquitin chains or by monoubiquitination or multimonoubiquitination, via an enzymatic cascade involving ubiquitin-activating E1, ubiquitin-conjugating E2 and ubiquitin-ligase E3. Protein polyubiquitination frequently leads to recognition by the 26S proteasome system and proteolytic processing. Gli1 undergoes, SCF/bTrCP/Skp1/Cullin1 ubiquitin-dependent degradation and this process controls tumor formation. A distinct mechanism has also been described to proteolytically process Gli via a different Cullin-based ligase (Cullin3). Cullin3 requires proteins containing a BTB domain to target substrates. One of these BTB proteins has been recently identified in *Drosophila* (HIB/Roadskill) and mouse (SPOP) [21].

We have recently reported a novel mechanism of switch-off of the Hedgehog pathway output involving the ubiquitination and degradation of Gli1 by Itch/AIP4, an additional E3 ubiquitin ligase belonging to a distinct HECT family [20]. This process is triggered by Numb. Indeed, Numb p66 isoform binds both Gli1 and Itch thus recruiting the E3 ligase activity and diverting Gli1 to a protein degradative pathway [20]. In this way, Numb suppresses Hedgehog signals and growth and promotes cell differentiation of cerebellar GCPs and medulloblastomas. Interestingly, Gli1 ubiquitination and degradation is reduced in human medulloblastoma due to the decreased levels of Numb and the consequent reduction of the activity of the Numb/E3 ligase Itch complex [20].

Therefore, the Numb-induced targeting of Gli1 for Itch-dependent ubiquitination unveils a role for this mechanism in limiting the extent and the duration of Hedgehog signals which otherwise would maintain an undifferentiated pool of neural progenitor cells susceptible to malignant transformation. Instead, as a result of this antagonism, progenitor cells are allowed to fulfill their physiological differentiation program. Thus Numb behaves as a novel tumor suppressor whose reduced expression in medulloblastoma allows the expansion of cancer stem cells.

Conclusions

The understanding of genetic and epigenetic changes that sustain malignant transformation and progression is essential to identify targets that can be employed for innovative therapeutic strategies. In this regard, a variety of targeting therapeutic agents appears to be necessary, depending on the very diverse disrupted cell functions that need to be rescued in cancer cells. While surgery remains a fundamental therapy, a rational treatment approach also requires a combination of cytotoxic chemotherapy and radiotherapy together with additional strategies (including gene therapy and drug-based targeting) addressing specific misregulated molecular events underlying the subverted biological processes of cancer cells. Although several hallmarks of cancer cell (e.g. uncontrolled cell proliferation, survival, invasiveness) need to be targeted, the most challenging task appears to be the eradication of cancer stem cells, which constitute a tiny minority of the tumor cell population. The elucidation of their biology is critical for designing appropriate agents able to control stemness cell identity.

References

1. Hahn WC, Weinberg RA (2002) Modelling the molecular circuitry of cancer. Nat Rev Cancer 2(5):331–341
2. Chin L, Gray JW (2008) Translating insights from the cancer genome into clinical practice. Nature 452(7187):553–563
3. Giannini G, Ristori E, Cerignoli F et al (2002) Human MRE11 is inactivated in mismatch repair-deficient cancers. EMBO Rep 3(3):248–254
4. Capalbo C, Buffone A, Vestri A et al (2007) Does the search for large genomic rearrangements impact BRCAPRO carrier prediction? J Clin Oncol 25(18):2632–2634
5. Palma M, Ristori E, Ricevuto E et al (2006) BRCA1 and BRCA2: the genetic testing and the current management options for mutation carriers. Crit Rev Oncol Hematol 57(1):1–23
6. Minucci S, Pelicci PG (2006) Histone deacetylase inhibitors and the promise of epigenetic (and more) treatments for cancer. Nat Rev Cancer 6:38–51
7. Tacconelli A, Farina AR, Cappabianca L et al (2004) TrkA alternative splicing: a regulated tumor-promoting switch in human neuroblastoma. Cancer Cell 6(4):347–360
8. Ferretti E, Di Marcotullio L, Gessi M et al (2006) Alternative splicing of the ErbB-4 cytoplasmic domain and its regulation by hedgehog signaling identify distinct medulloblastoma subsets. Oncogene 25(55):7267–7273
9. Bellavia D, Mecarozzi M, Campese AF et al (2007) Notch3 and the Notch3-upregulated RNA-binding protein HuD regulate Ikaros alternative splicing. EMBO J.; 26(6):1670–1680
10. Calin GA, Croce CM (2006) MicroRNA signatures in human cancers. Nat Rev Cancer 6:857–866
11. Laneve P, Di Marcotullio L, Gioia U et al (2007) The interplay between microRNAs and the neurotrophin receptor tropomyosin-related kinase C controls proliferation of human neuroblastoma cells. Proc Natl Acad Sci U S A 104:7957–7962
12. Ruiz i Altaba A (2006) Hedgehog-Gli signaling in human diseases. Ed Landes Bioscience, Kluwer Academic/Plenum Publishers, New York
13. Ferretti E, De Smaele E, Di Marcotullio L et al (2005) Hedgehog checkpoints in medulloblastoma: the chromosome 17p deletion paradigm. Trends Mol Med 11(12):537–545

14. Thompson MC, Fuller C, Hogg TL et al (2006) Genomics identifies medulloblastoma subgroups that are enriched for specific genetic alterations. J Clin Oncol 24:1924–1931
15. Gallo R, Zazzeroni F, Alesse E et al (2002) REN: a novel, developmentally regulated gene that promotes neural cell differentiation. J Cell Biol 158(4):731–740
16. Argenti B, Gallo R, Di Marcotullio L et al (2005) Hedgehog antagonist REN(KCTD11) regulates proliferation and apoptosis of developing granule cell progenitors. J Neurosci 25(36):8338–8346
17. Di Marcotullio L, Ferretti E, De Smaele E et al (2004) REN(KCTD11) is a suppressor of Hedgehog signaling and is deleted in human medulloblastoma. Proc Natl Acad Sci U S A 101(29):10833–10838
18. Di Marcotullio L, Ferretti E, De Smaele E et al (2006) Suppressors of hedgehog signaling: Linking aberrant development of neural progenitors and tumorigenesis. Mol Neurobiol 34(3):193–204
19. Singh SK, Hawkins C, Clarke ID et al (2004) Identification of human brain tumour initiating cells. Nature 432:396–401
20. Di Marcotullio L, Ferretti E, Greco A et al (2006) Numb is a suppressor of Hedgehog signalling and targets Gli1 for Itch-dependent ubiquitination. Nat Cell Biol 8(12):1415-1423
21. Di Marcotullio L, Ferretti E, Greco A et al (2007) Multiple ubiquitin-dependent processing pathways regulate hedgehog/gli signaling: implications for cell development and tumorigenesis. Cell Cycle 6(4):390-393
22. Klein AL, Zilian O, Suter U, Taylor V (2004) Murine numb regulates granule cell maturation in the cerebellum. Dev Biol 266(1):161–177

Chapter 4

The Medical Oncologist's Point of View

Massimo Lopez, Laura Giacinti, Silvia I.S. Fattoruso

In the treatment of cancer, one of the basic assumptions is that all malignant cells should be removed or destroyed to achieve cure. To do this, surgery and/or radiotherapy have been traditionally the primary chosen treatments in solid tumors. However, neither modality can be considered curative once disease is beyond the local region, and clinical evidence has already shown that surgical removal or radiotherapeutic ablation of "localized" masses do not achieve the desired cancer control in a large number of patients. In fact, many tumors which are apparently localized are already microscopically disseminated.

If disseminated disease exists at the time of diagnosis, then some therapeutic approach is needed which has the ability to kill tumor cells anywhere in the body. Chemotherapy has been the master candidate for adjuvant use to local therapy, and has considerably contributed to the development of one of the most important achievements in the strategy of cancer treatment, namely the combined modality approach. For a long time the pediatric oncologist has been aware of the value of multimodal treatment because of the results initially obtained in Wilms' tumor, embryonal rhabdomyosarcoma, Ewing's sarcoma, and osteogenic sarcoma. This potential, however, has come to be appreciated also by the clinical oncologist treating breast cancer and other major cancer killers.

The development of this strategy requires a multidisciplinary input at least from surgical oncologists, radiation oncologists, medical oncologists and pathologists. The role of medical oncologists has became increasingly important as more new effective drugs have been clinically available and, more recently, with the coming of age of molecular-targeted agents.

We are in an exciting period of therapeutic research in which the potential to increase the control of several malignancies is high. If we are to fulfil this potential we will need to exploit even more fully the multidisciplinary approach to a disease-oriented strategy. No longer can any single therapeutic modality consider itself as the sole treatment of cancer, although some priorities need to be set especially when the unlimited numbers of interaction occurring with combined modality treatment are considered. At any rate, multimodal cooperation should today be the routine approach to cancer treatment [1].

A. Bolognese, L. Izzo (eds.), *Surgery in Multimodal Management of Solid Tumors.*
©Springer-Verlag Italia 2009

There are several examples of how the multimodality approach may be applied for optimal patient management. A few are reported here, including colorectal cancer and liver metastases from this disease, gastric cancer, and pancreatic cancer.

Colorectal Cancer

The management of colorectal cancer has changed dramatically over the last 25 years due to advances in chemotherapy, surgery, and radiotherapy.

For many years, the cornerstone of systemic treatment for advanced colon cancer was fluorouracil (FU), whose clinical activity could be improved with leucovorin (LV) modulation (Table 4.1). This led to an evaluation of combined FU and LV in the adjuvant setting, where it was found to improve disease-free survival (DFS) and overall survival (OS) in patients with Stage III disease [2].

A significant increase in therapeutic results was obtained with the development of newer cytotoxic agents, such as irinotecan, oxaliplatin and capecitabine, and several monoclonal antibodies (MoAb), including cetuximab, bevacizumab and panitumumab. While the addition of irinotecan to FU and LV in the treatment of patients with resected Stage II or III colon cancer did not result in a meaningful improvement in outcome [3, 4], a statistically significant benefit was observed with the use of oxaliplatin.

The European MOSAIC trial evaluated the efficacy of FOLFOX4 (infusional fluorouracil, leucovorin, oxaliplatin) compared to infusional FU/LV in 2,246 patients with completely resected Stage II or Stage III colon cancer. After a median follow-up of 49 months, the 4-year DFS in patients with Stage III disease was statistically superior in those patients who received oxaliplatin (69.7% vs. 61%) [5, 6]. A significant improvement was not observed in Stage II disease, although a 5.4% absolute increase in DFS was noted in patients at high-risk, including the presence of T4 tumor stage, bowel obstruction, tumor perforation, poorly differentiated histology, venous invasion, or <10 examined lymph nodes. These results were later confirmed by NSABP C-07 trial, which randomized 2,407 patients with resected Stage II or Stage III colon cancer to receive bolus FU/LV with or without oxaliplatin [7].

Single agent capecitabine, an oral prodrug of fluorouracil, as adjuvant therapy for patients with Stage III colon cancer was also shown to be similarly effective when compared with monthly bolus FU/LV [8], and another study, known as the XELOXA trial, randomized 1,886 patients with resected Stage III colon cancer to receive either capecitabine and oxaliplatin or bolus FU/LV [9]. At present, efficacy results from this study are not available.

All these studies have considerably enriched the treatment options for patients with Stage III resected colon cancer. The combination of fluorouracil, leucovorin and oxaliplatin for 6 months is considered the standard of care because it seems more effective in comparison to other fluorouracil-based treatments. However, in some instances, either single agent capecitabine or FU/LV may be appropriate adjuvant treatments.

Table 4.1 Chemotherapy regimens in advanced colorectal cancer

Regimen	Chemotherapy dosing	Schedule
Fluoropyrimidines		
Roswell Park	FU 500 mg/m^2 bolus LV 500 mg/m^2 over 2 hours	Weekly for 6 of 8 weeks
Mayo Clinic	FU 425 mg/m^2 bolus on days 1 to 5 LV 20 mg/m^2 bolus on days 1 to 5	Every 4 to 5 weeks
Capecitabine	1250 mg/m^2 orally twice daily on days 1 to 14	Every 3 weeks
Irinotecan		
IFL	FU 500 mg/m^2 bolus LV 20 mg/m^2 bolus Irinotecan 125 mg/m^2	Weekly for 4 of 6 weeks
FOLFIRI	FU 400 mg/m^2 bolus on day 1 + 2400–3000 mg/m^2 c.i. over 46 hours on days 1 and 2 LV 400 mg/m^2 over 2 hours on day 1 Irinotecan 180 mg/m^2 on day 1	Every 2 weeks
Oxaliplatin		
FOLFOX4	FU 400 mg/m^2 bolus + 600 mg/m^2 c.i. over 22 hours on days 1 and 2 LV 200 mg/m^2 over 2 hours on days 1 and 2 Oxaliplatin 85 mg/m^2 on day 1	Every 2 weeks
CapeOX	Oxaliplatin 130 mg/m^2 day 1 Capecitabine 850-1000 mg/m^2 twice daily for 14 days	Every 3 weeks
Cetuximab + irinotecan	Cetuximab 250 mg/m^2 on days 1 and 8 (first dose only: 400 mg/m^2) Irinotecan 180 mg/m^2 on day 1	Every 2 weeks
Bevacizumab + FU based-regimens	Bevacizumab 5 mg/kg on day 1 + FU/LV (Roswell Park) or FOLFOX or FOLFIRI or CapeOX	Every 2 weeks

FU, Fluoracil; *LV*, leucovorin; *c.i.*, continuous intravenous infusion

In Stage II colon cancer, no single randomized clinical trial has yet demonstrated a survival benefit for adjuvant therapy. Thus, this treatment remains controversial, but evidence has accumulated suggesting that it should be considered in patients with poor prognostic features [10].

The close proximity of the rectum to pelvic structures, the absence of a serosa surrounding the rectum, and technical difficulties associated with achieving wide negative margins are all factors determining a relatively high risk of local recurrence in patients with rectal cancer. Combined-modality therapy of this disease is, therefore, somewhat different from that of colon cancer, including differences in surgical technique, the use of radiotherapy, and the method of chemotherapy administration.

More than two decades ago, the results of a Gastrointestinal Tumor Study Group (GITSG) and a subsequent North Central Cancer Treatment Group (NCCTG) randomized trials demonstrated a statistically significant reduction in the rate of local recurrence and an increase in DFS and OS when long-course radiation was administered concurrently with intravenous FU after surgical resection for patients with Stage II or III rectal cancer. Adjuvant chemoradiotherapy became, therefore, the standard of care in all patients with completely resected Stage II or III rectal cancer. It was also reported that postoperative radiotherapy given concurrently with infusional FU was associated with improved local control and survival compared with bolus FU and radiation.

More recently, a new standard of care has emerged due to the results of the German Rectal Cancer Study, which directly compared preoperative versus postoperative chemoradiotherapy in 823 patients with clinical Stage II or III rectal cancer [11]. Patients randomized to preoperative treatment received 50.4 Gy in 28 fractions with a 120-hour infusion of FU at 1000 mg/m^2/day during the first and fifth weeks of radiation. One month after surgery, including total mesorectal excision (TME), they received adjuvant chemotherapy, consisting of 4 cycles of bolus FU at 500 mg/m^2/day for 5 days every 4 weeks (Mayo Clinic regimen). Patients randomized to initial surgery received the same chemoradiation and subsequent FU postoperatively, with the exception of an additional radiation boost (5.4 Gy) to the tumor bed. Preoperative chemoradiation doubled the rate of sphincter-sparing operations and lowered the rates of local recurrence and toxicity. However, no difference in DFS and OS was observed between the two treatment groups (Table 4.2).

For patients with Stage II or III rectal cancer, available data support the use of concurrent radiotherapy and continuous infusion FU, and resection performed by TME. Neoadjuvant chemoradiotherapy and subsequent surgery are typically followed by 4 months of adjuvant chemotherapy.

Currently, randomized data are not available to support the use of capecitabine, irinotecan, or oxaliplatin in the adjuvant treatment of rectal cancer. Nevertheless, FOLFOX and capecitabine may be considered in this setting, mostly as an extrapolation from the data available from colon cancer.

Over the last 5 years, molecularly targeted agents have increased the therapeutic armamentarium in patients with metastatic colorectal cancer, with increased chances of prolonged survival. We can now select from three different MoAb, targeting either the epidermal growth factor receptor (EGFR) or vascular endothelial growth factor (VEGF). The role of these MoAb in the adjuvant treatment of colon cancer (Table 4.3) and rectal cancer (Table 4.4) has not yet been defined, but several clinical trials are ongoing in this setting.

Table 4.2 Results of the German Rectal Cancer Study of Postoperative Versus Preoperative Chemoradiation in Stage II and III Rectal Cancer

Treatment arm	Local recurrence	Disease-free survival	Overall survival	Sphincter-sparing surgery	G_{3-4} acute toxicity	G_{3-4} long-term toxicity
Preoperative (%)	6	68	76	39	27	14
Postoperative (%)	13	65	74	19	40	24
p value	0.006	0.32	0.80	0.004	0.001	0.01

Survival and recurrence rates were determined at 5 years

Table 4.3 Ongoing clinical trials in adjuvant treatment of colon cancer

Trial	AJCC stage	Randomization
NCCTG N0147	III	FOLFOX versus FOLFOX + cetuximab
PETACC-8	III	FOLFOX versus FOLFOX + cetuximab
NSABP C-08	II, III	FOLFOX versus FOLFOX + bevacizumab
AVANT	II, III	FOLFOX versus FOLFOX + bevacizumab versus capecitabine + oxaliplatin + bevacizumab
ECOG E5202	II	Molecular high risk: FOLFOX versus FOLFOX + bevacizumab

NCCTG, North Central Cancer Treatment Group; *PETACC*, Pan European Trials in Adjuvant Colon Cancer; *NSABP*, National Surgical Adjuvant Breast and Bowel Project; *AVANT*, International Phase III study of bevacizumab, XELOX, and FOLFOX chemotherapy regimens in early-stage colon cancer; *ECOG*, Eastern Cooperative Oncology Group; *FOLFOX*, fluorouracil, leucovorin, and oxaliplatin

Table 4.4 Ongoing clinical trials in adjuvant treatment of rectal cancer

Trial	Setting	Randomization
NSABP R-04	Preoperative chemoradiation without oxaliplatin	FU versus capecitabine with or
Accord-12	Preoperative chemoradiation + oxaliplatin	Capecitabine versus capecitabine
RTOG 0247	Preoperative chemoradiation	Capecitabine and irinotecan versus capecitabine and oxaliplatin
French Intergroup R98	Adjuvant chemotherapy	FU/LV versus FU/LV/irinotecan
US Gastrointestinal Intergroup	Adjuvant chemotherapy	FU/LV/oxaliplatin versus FU/LV/oxaliplatin/bevacizumab

NSABP, National Surgical Adjuvant Breast and Bowel Project; *RTOG*, Radiation Therapy Oncology Group; *FU*, fluorouracil; *LV*, leucovorin

Overall, in patients with potentially resectable tumors, advances in surgery, radiation and chemotherapy have all contributed to increase cure rates. In patients with metastatic disease, the incorporation of new cytotoxic drugs and molecularly targeted agents has led to an increase in median overall survival from less than 9 months without treatment to greater than 20 months [12]. However, the only chance to cure patients with metastatic colorectal cancer is the possibility of resection of metastatic disease. Typically, the 5-year survival rates following resection of liver-only metastases range from 25 to 35% [13], but only 10-20% of patients are eligible for liver surgery [14].

Although a large body of evidence has demonstrated that liver resection is safe and effective, the concept of resectability has evolved lasting recent years, and frequently surgeon faces borderline cases. In this scenario, chemotherapy may have an important role to play within a multimodal approach.

Patients with initially unresectable metastases that are downsized to resectable metastases by chemotherapy have a chance of long-term survival similar to that of patients with liver metastases deemed resectable from the outset. In these cases, surgery should be performed as soon as liver metastases become resectable, to avoid tumor progression during systemic treatment. In addition, it is important to avoid complete clinical response, since a microscopic residue of disease remains in most of the sites, which are considered to have disappeared on imaging [15]. Resection of the site of initial metastases is necessary, and attention should be paid to carefully identify the precise site of resection and to achieve a sufficient resection margin.

Although there are no compelling data to support pretreatment with neoadjuvant chemotherapy in patients with resectable liver metastases, preoperative systemic therapy may be an option because it offers the possibility to test the chemosensitivity of the tumor to a specific therapeutic regimen, and to eradicate microscopic foci of disease that may contribute to recurrence after surgery.

In dealing with systemic treatment, it is important to determine the combination of cytotoxic and molecular agents with the highest likelihood of inducing a response. Currently, bevacizumab combined with FOLFIRI (fluorouracil, leucovorin, irinotecan), FOLFOX or CapeOX (capecitabine, oxaliplatin) may be an appropriate choice. Several new studies are evaluating the proportion of patients that will undergo resection after downsizing of initially unresectable liver metastases while being treated with chemotherapy in combination with one or two targeted agents. At any rate, safety evaluation is important because of uncertainty about the impact of angiogenesis inhibitors on postoperative complications, wound healing, and liver regeneration.

Gastric Cancer

Although in the past gastric cancer was considered for a long time the most chemosensitive tumor of the gastrointestinal tract, only recently has chemotherapy been definitively incorporated in the multimodality treatment of this disease.

Adjuvant chemotherapy in gastric cancer has been studied extensively during the past four decades, but definitive conclusions from randomized trials cannot be drawn because only rarely has significant improved survival been observed. Initial meta-analyses concluded that postoperative chemotherapy did not add a survival benefit to surgery. A slightly significant benefit of adjuvant systemic therapy was found in other meta-analyses [16], but these results have not generally influenced standard clinical practice.

Postoperative chemoradiation was established mainly in the USA following the results of the landmark trial INT-0116 [17]. Patients with T3 and/or node positive adenocarcinoma of the stomach or gastroesophageal junction, after resection with negative margins were randomized to either observation alone or combined modality therapy consisting of 5 monthly cycles of bolus FU/LV with radiotherapy (45 Gy) concurrent with cycles 2 and 3. There was a significant decrease in local failure (19% vs. 29%), as well as an increase in median survival (36 vs. 27 months) and OS (50% vs. 41%, $p=0.005$) with combined modality treatment.

Among several combination chemotherapy regimens used in advanced gastric cancer (Table 4.5), a Cochrane review found the best survival rates with anthracyclines, cisplatin and FU [18]. The regimen ECF (epirubicin, cisplatin, infusional FU), which proved to be the best tolerated, was therefore used in perioperative chemotherapy by the British Medical Research Council in the MAGIC study [19]. Patients with resectable adenocarcinoma of the stomach or gastroesophageal junction were randomized to receive either perioperative chemother-

Table 4.5 Chemotherapy regimens in advanced gastric cancer

FP	FU 1000 mg/m^2 c.i. on days 1 to 5 DDP 100 mg/m^2 on day 1	Every 4 weeks
ECF	Epirubicin 50 mg/m^2 on day 1 DDP 60 mg/m^2 on day 1 FU 200 mg/m^2 c.i. on days 1 to 21	Every 3 weeks
ECX	Epirubicin 50 mg/m^2 on day 1 DDP 60 mg/m^2 on day 1 Capecitabine 1000 mg/m^2 twice daily on days 1 to 14	Every 3 weeks
DCF	Docetaxel 75 mg/m^2 on day 1 DDP 75 mg/m^2 on day 1 FU 750 mg/m^2/day c.i. 24 h on days 1 to 5	Every 3 weeks
FLO	FU 2600 mg/m^2 c.i. 24 h Oxaliplatin 85 mg/m^2 on day 1 LV 200 mg/m^2 on day 1	Every 2 weeks

c.i., Continuous intravenous infusion; *DDP*, cisplatin; *FU*, fluorouracil; *LV*, leucovorin apy (three preoperative and three postoperative cycles of ECF) or surgery alone. Five-year survival rates were 36% among those who received perioperative chemotherapy and 23% in the surgery group. The main drawback of ECF is the continuous infusion FU, which requires long-term intravenous access and an infusion pump.

Similar results have been recently reported by the French FFCD (*Fédération Française de Cancérologie Digestive*) Group study in patients with resectable adenocarcinoma of the stomach randomized to receive surgery alone or 2–3 cycles of preoperative FP (infusional FU, cisplatin). Postoperative FP was recommended in case of response to FP preoperative or stable disease with pN+ [20].

Currently, after decades of negative studies, two successful strategies in localized gastric cancer are available. Like postoperative chemoradiation, perioperative chemotherapy should also be considered a standard treatment option for patients with resectable gastric cancer. Nevertheless, there is no evidence to suggest that either perioperative or postoperative chemoradiotherapy is superior. Probably, the preferred strategy will be chosen by the referral patterns that are prevalent in a given center. For perioperative chemotherapy to be feasible, patients must be referred to an oncologist prior to surgery and a multidisciplinary team should discuss all new patients.

Notwithstanding these achievements, there is an urgent need for more active and more practical combined modality treatments. Ongoing and proposed studies will assess the role of a potentially more active postoperative chemoradiation regimen (Intergroup study, Cancer and Leukemia Group B 80101), the role of adding bevacizumab to perioperative chemotherapy (MAGIC-B, using ECX regimen, with capecitabine instead of infusional FU), and the role of postoperative chemoradiation in combination with preoperative chemotherapy (CRITICS study by the Dutch Gastric Cancer Group).

Pancreatic Cancer

Currently, more than 80% of patients with pancreatic cancer present with disease that cannot be cured by surgical treatment, underscoring the need for additional modalities to improve on therapeutic results. Unfortunately, progress in the systemic treatment of pancreatic adenocarcinoma did not occur for several decades, and only in recent years could some new drugs be added to fluorouracil.

Adjuvant chemotherapy has been reported effective in the ESPAC-1 trial which assigned patients at random to chemotherapy (bolus FU/LV given on 5 days for six 28-day cycles) or no chemotherapy, and radiotherapy or no radiotherapy [21]. The 5-year survival rate was 10% in patients receiving chemoradiotherapy and 20% in those who did not receive this treatment ($p = 0.05$), whereas it was 21% in patients who received chemotherapy and 8% in those who did not receive systemic treatment ($p = 0.009$). Thus, these provocative results suggest that FU is superior to observation and that chemoradiotherapy is unnecessary and perhaps harmful in patients with resected pancreatic cancer.

Recently, the results from the large phase III CONKO-001 trial have been published. This study randomized 368 patients with resected pancreatic cancer to observation or gemcitabine for six cycles of 4 weeks. Gemcitabine had been reported to be superior to bolus FU in metastatic pancreatic cancer, but has only limited antitumor efficacy in measurable disease, with an objective response rate of less than 10% and a median survival of less than 6 months. In the adjuvant setting, DFS was 13.4 months in the gemcitabine group and 6.9 months in the control group (p <0.001) [22]. However, no difference in OS was observed in the two groups (22.1 months in the gemcitabine arm and 20.2 months in the control group; p = 0.061). Despite the absence of radiation, the benefit from chemotherapy was observed both in patients with R0 and R1 resections.

The RTOG 97-04 trial randomly allocated over 500 patients to a 3-week course of chemotherapy (protracted infusion FU 250 mg/m^2/day versus gemcitabine 1000 mg/m^2 once), then chemoradiotherapy (50.4 Gy and protracted infusion FU), and then a 3-month course of chemotherapy with the same drugs as in the pre-chemoradiotherapy course [23]. In patients with tumors of the pancreas head, results of this study showed a 3-year survival rate of 32% in the gemcitabine group compared with 21% in the FU group (p = 0.033). However, when all patients in the study were included, no significant survival differences were observed.

Although a comparison between these three randomized trials cannot be made because of differences in the treatment design and patient characteristics, it is noteworthy that median OS for patients treated with gemcitabine (22.1 months in the CONKO-001 trial and 20.6 months in the RTOG 97-04 trial) and bolus FU (20.1 months in the ESPAC-1 trial) was remarkably similar. Thus, at this time, several choices are available for adjuvant treatment of pancreatic adenocarcinoma: FU-based chemoradiotherapy with additional gemcitabine chemotherapy and chemotherapy alone with gemcitabine, FU or capecitabine. The substitution of this agent for infusional or bolus FU is generally considered appropriate, especially because of a favorable toxicity profile.

Since uncertainty remains about the best adjuvant chemotherapy to use, a new study (ESPAC-3) has been designed which randomizes patients to receive either FU/LV (as used in the ESPAC-1 trial) or gemcitabine (a third observation arm was stopped after the definitive results of the ESPAC-1 trial).

As with gastric carcinoma, it could be hypothesized that chemotherapy would be more useful before surgery than after surgery. In fact, there is some evidence that more patients with resectable pancreatic adenocarcinoma may benefit from preoperative therapy, because the prolonged recovery after pancreaticoduodenectomy prevents the delivery of postoperative therapy in up to 25% of the eligible patients. Several studies have investigated the use of neoadjuvant chemoradiotherapy in patients with resectable disease but, to date, there is no randomized trial addressing this issue. Thus, the use of neoadjuvant therapy outside of a clinical trial in patients with clinically resectable disease is not supported by available data.

Some studies have tested the use of preoperative chemoradiation treatment to convert an unresectable disease to a resectable one. Although preoperative therapy has resulted in a better chance of a margin-negative resection, no randomized trial involving R0 resection rate as endpoint has yet been reported. In this regard, it should be considered that single agent or combination chemotherapy regimens are not available that result in a high percentage of good clinical responses in advanced disease.

Phase II trial results of gemcitabine with new targeted agents (eg, bevacizumab, cetuximab, erlotinib) have been encouraging in patients with advanced pancreatic cancer, but only the combination of gemcitabine and erlotinib was associated with a statistically significant increase in survival when compared to gemcitabine alone in a phase III trial [24]. Nevertheless, this improvement was clinically modest, and objective response rates were not significantly different between the two arms, being 8.6% with erlotinib and gemcitabine and 8.0% with placebo and gemcitabine.

In the search for newer and more effective therapies in patients with pancreatic adenocarcinoma, however, adjuvant clinical trials incorporating principles of molecular biology should be considered. Although ineffective in combination with cytotoxic agents, bevacizumab and cetuximab may play a role as radiosensitizers, and new targets are being evaluated for therapeutic development [25]. One of these is nuclear factor-kappa B (NF-kB), a transcription factor that is constitutively activated in pancreatic cancer. NF-kB has been targeted using curcumin, a natural product with promising activity in a pilot clinical trial [26]. Several other targeted agents are under investigation in pancreatic cancer, but a greater understanding of molecular biology of this disease is of paramount importance to better exploit the therapeutic potential of molecularly targeted drugs.

References

1. Niederhuber JE (2004) Surgical intervention in cancer. In: Abeloff MD, Armitage JO, Niederhuber JE, Kastan MB, McKenna WG (eds) Clinical Oncology, 3rd edn. Elsevier, Philadelphia, pp 579–590
2. Gill S, Loprinzi CL, Sargent DJ et al (2004) Pooled analysis of fluorouracil-based adjuvant therapy for stage II and III colon cancer: who benefits and by how much? J Clin Oncol 22:1797–1806
3. Saltz LB, Niedzwiecki D, Hollis D et al (2004) Irinotecan plus fluorouracil/leucovorin (IFL) versus fluorouracil/leucovorin (FL) in stage III colon cancer (intergroup trial CALGB C89803). Proc Am Soc Clin Oncol 22:246s
4. Van Cutsem E, Labianca R, Hossfeld G et al (2005) Randomized phase III trial comparing infused irinotecan/5-fluorouracil (5-FU)/folinic acid (IF) versus 5-FU/FA (F) in stage III colon cancer patients (PETACC 3). J Clin Oncol 23:3s
5. Andre T, Boni C, Mounedji-Boudiaf L et al (2004) Oxaliplatin, fluorouracil, and leucovorin as adjuvant treatment for colon cancer. N Engl J Med 350:2343–2351
6. De Gramont A, Boni C, Navarro M et al (2005) Oxaliplatin/5FU/LV in the adjuvant treatment of stage II and stage III colon cancer: efficacy results with a median follow-up of 4 years. Proc Am Soc Clin Oncol 23:246s

7. Wolmark N, Wieand HS, Keubler JP et al (2005) A phase III trial comparing FULV to FULV + oxaliplatin in stage II or III carcinoma of the colon: results of NSABP protocol C-07. J Clin Oncol 23:16s

8. Twelves C, Wong A, Nowacki MP et al (2005) Capecitabine as adjuvant treatment for stage III colon cancer. N Engl J Med 352:2696–2704

9. Schmoll H, Tabernero J, Nowacki M et al (2005) Early safety findings from a phase III trial of capecitabine plus oxaliplatin (XELOX) vs. bolus 5-FU/LV as adjuvant therapy for patients with stage III colon cancer. J Clin Oncol 23:16s

10. Benson AB III, Schrag D, Somerfield MR et al (2004) American Society of Clinical Oncology recommendations on adjuvant chemotherapy for stage II colon cancer. J Clin Oncol 22:3408–3419

11. Sauer R, Becker H, Hohenberger W et al (2004) Preoperative versus postoperative chemoradiotherapy for rectal cancer. N Engl J Med 351:1731–1740

12. Meyerhardt JA, Mayer RJ (2005) Systemic therapy for colorectal cancer. N Engl J Med 352:476–487

13. Fong Y, Cohen AM, Fortner JG et al (1997) Liver resection for colorectal metastases. J Clin Oncol 15:938–946

14. Modern multimodality approach to hepatic colorectal metastases: solutions and controversies (2007) Surg Oncol 16:71–83

15. Benoist S, Brouquet A, Penna C (2006) Complete response of colorectal liver metastases after chemotherapy: does it mean cure? J Clin Oncol 24:3939–3945

16. Zhao SL, Fang JY (2008) The role of postoperative adjuvant chemotherapy following curative resection for gastric cancer: a meta-analysis. Cancer Invest 26:317–325

17. Macdonald JS, Smalley SR, Benedetti J et al (2001) Chemoradiotherapy after surgery compared with surgery alone for adenocarcinoma of the stomach or gastroesophageal junction. N Engl J Med 345:725–730

18. Wagner AD, Grothe W, Haerting J, et al (2006) Chemotherapy in advanced gastric cancer: a systematic review and meta-analysis based on aggregate data. J Clin Oncol 24:2903–2909

19. Cunningham D, Allum WH, Stenning SP et al (2006) Perioperative chemotherapy versus surgery alone for resectable gastroesophageal cancer. N Engl J Med 355:11–20

20. Boige V, Pignon J, Saint-Aubert B et al (2007) Final results of a randomized trial comparing preoperative 5-fluorouracil (F)/cisplatin (P) to surgery alone in adenocarcinoma of stomach and lower esophagus (ASLE): FNLCC ACCORD07-FFCD 9703 trial. J Clin Oncol 25:18s

21. Neoptolemos JP, Stocken DD, Friess H et al (2004) A randomized trial of chemoradiotherapy and chemotherapy after resection of pancreatic cancer. N Engl J Med 350:1200–1210

22. Oettle H, Post S, Neuhaus P et al (2007) Adjuvant chemotherapy with gemcitabine vs. observation in patients undergoing curative-intent resection of pancreatic cancer: a randomized controlled trial. JAMA 297:267–277

23. Regine WF, Abrams RA (2006) Adjuvant therapy for pancreatic cancer: current status, future directions. Semin Oncol 33:S10-S13

24. Moore MJ, Goldstein D, Hamm J et al (2007) Erlotinib plus gemcitabine compared with gemcitabine alone in patients with advanced pancreatic cancer: a phase III trial of the National Cancer Institute of Canada Clinical Trials Group. J Clin Oncol 25:1960–1966

25. Abbruzzese J, Kurzrock R, McConkey D et al (2007) Are there rational novel targets for pancreatic cancer terapeutics? Observation from the MD Anderson Cancer Center SPORE in pancreatic cancer. Eur J Cancer 5:149

26. Li L, Aggarwal BB, Shishodia S et al (2004) Nuclear factor-kappaB and IkappaB kinase are constitutively active in human pancreatic cells, and their down-regulation by curcumin (diferuloylmethane) is associated with the suppression of proliferation and the induction of apoptosis. Cancer 101:2351–2362

Chapter 5

The Radiotherapist's Point of View

Riccardo Maurizi Enrici, Mattia F. Osti, Francesca Berardi

Radiotherapy has played a central role in the treatment of neoplasms since the discovery of X-rays, particularly with regard to organ preservation where mutilating procedures may be avoided.

Radiotherapy may have a curative or symptomatic intent. It can be used alone or in association with other therapies such as surgery and/or chemotherapy or radio sensitizer, radio protectors, whether immunological or biological.

Combined modalities therapy is today the gold standard for treatment of the most common tumors. In this report we will briefly consider the role of radiation therapy in the multimodalities approach to gastrointestinal cancers.

Radiotherapy in Cancer of the Esophagus

The treatment of choice for carcinoma of the esophagus is surgery. Nevertheless, considering the high rate of late diagnosis and high incidence of recurrence, even after radical surgery adjuvant treatment is required. Radiotherapy (RT), performed exclusively in alternative to surgery produces modest results, inferior to those of surgery. The most important studies carried out in the past reported locoregional relapse rates of around 70–80% after doses of 56–61 Gy and a 2-year survival rate of 10 to 20% and a 5-year survival rate of 2%. Thus, in light of the results obtained by multimodal treatments, there is a wide consensus that radiotherapy alone must be reserved only for patients unfit for combined treatments.

In recent years, numerous trials have used radiotherapy with concomitant chemotherapy (RT-CHT), both as a single, adjuvant or neoadjuvant treatment. In the RTOG 85-01 trial, 121 patients were randomized to receive 50 Gy + 5-FU + CDDP vs. RT alone (64 Gy). Results showed a 5 year survival rate of 27% for patients in the group of combined therapy, vs. 0% in the radiotherapy alone group. Median survival was also better for the first group (14.1 months vs. 9.3 months) [1]. These results suggest that chemoradiotherapy is the best option and dose escalation does not determine a survival benefit.

In the Intergroup trial 0122, radiotherapy and chemotherapy were intensified. The study reported a higher treatment-related mortality rate (9% vs. 2%) and no local control improvement compared to the RTOG 85-01.

A. Bolognese, L. Izzo (eds.), *Surgery in Multimodal Management of Solid Tumors.*
©Springer-Verlag Italia 2009

Data reported by Minsky also confirmed that higher doses do not increase survival or local control; in fact, in a series of 236 patients, 109 were submitted to combined treatment with CDDP, 5-FU and RT with 64.8 Gy; 127 patients were instead treated with the same chemotherapy and a dose of 50.4 Gy. The median survival time was 13 months vs. 18 months and the 2 year survival rate was 31% vs. 40%, respectively [2]. These data were not statistically significant.

Hyper-fractionated schemes have been investigated with the purpose of comparing this treatment to standard schedules. Zhao treated 56 patients with 41.4 Gy in 5 weeks, followed by 2 weeks of radiation at 3 Gy per day, with 2 sessions of 1.5 Gy, 6 hours apart. Total dose ranged between 67 and 70 Gy. The results were encouraging with a 5-year local control of 85% [3]. Yu reported encouraging results with a local control of 94% with combined chemotherapy (cisplatin and 5-FU during weeks 1, 4 and 7) and hyper-fractionated radiotherapy (1.8–2 Gy, twice daily during weeks 2, 5 and 8 reaching a total dose of 60 Gy); the results showed good local control but an elevated toxicity and a 30% mortality rate.

It is still unclear if a neoadjuvant therapeutic approach plus surgery is superior to surgery alone. Urba treated 100 patients randomized in two groups: the first underwent combined treatment with 5-FU + CDDP + Vinblastine and 45 Gy in two daily fractions of 1.5 Gy followed by surgery. The second group was submitted to surgery alone. After a median 8-year follow-up, the 3-year survival rate was better (32% vs. 16%) and the onset of local recurrence clearly inferior (19% vs. 30%) in the group submitted to neoadjuvant therapy but these findings were not statistically significant. Furthermore, findings showed that even in the absence of treatment-related mortality, patients submitted to combined therapy showed an 80% bone marrow toxicity of grade III–IV [4]. These data confirmed results obtained by Bosset et al in a randomized study which showed no advantage, in terms of survival, in patients treated with a neoadjuvant approach [5].

Different results were reported by Walsh in a randomized study in which the group submitted to concomitant chemoradiotherapy, followed by surgery, showed a total 3-year survival of 32% against the 6% of the group which received surgery alone ($p = 0.01$) [6].

Recently concomitant chemoradiotherapy followed by surgery was compared to chemoradiotherapy alone: in a randomized phase III study performed by Bonnetain et al, all patients received chemotherapy (5-FU + CDDP) and concomitant RT (46 Gy with standard fractioning). Subsequently, patients were randomly divided into two groups: the first underwent surgery while the second continued the combined treatment up to a total dose of 61 Gy. Results showed a 2-year survival rate of 40% vs. 34%, with a median survival of 19.3 vs. 17.7 months in favor of the non surgery group. Results were not statistically significant ($p = 0.88$) [7].

On the basis of this, it can be stated that radiochemotherapy alone is comparable to neoadjuvant radiochemotherapy followed by surgery. In inoperable patients, where the objective is palliation, radiotherapy handles symptoms in 60–80% of cases with doses of 30–50 Gy. Endocavitary brachitherapy administered at high (HDR) or low dose rate (LDR) is also useful in palliation. It is performed alone or in association with external beams. The best dose and fraction-ation have not been established yet. Harvey compared results of 22 patients treated with 20 Gy in 3 fractions LDR or 12/5 Gy in single fraction HDR; both therapies showed similar results [8].

Technical Notes on Radiotherapy

All patients undergo a CT scan with acquisition of the images from C5 till L1; slice thickness under 5 mm. To reduce set-up, patients are positioned with immobilization devices (Fig. 5.1).

For radical purposes the target is represented by the gross tumor volume (GTV) consisting of gross disease together with involved nodes. The clinical tar-get volume (CTV) includes the GTV plus 5 cm in the craniocaudal and 2 cm in the anteroposterior direction. In order to reduce toxicity and to increase dosages, large volumes are no longer used and only involved nodes are drawn. To get a better volume definition a PET-CT may prove useful. The administered doses are 55–60 Gy in cases of radiotherapy alone and 45–55 Gy in cases of combined chemoradiation.

Irradiation techniques are sophisticated due to the presence of organs at risk (OAR) such as the upper airways, the trachea, the lungs, the pleura, the heart and the bone marrow. The risk of acute and late toxicity is correlated with total and daily dose, dose per fraction and volume.

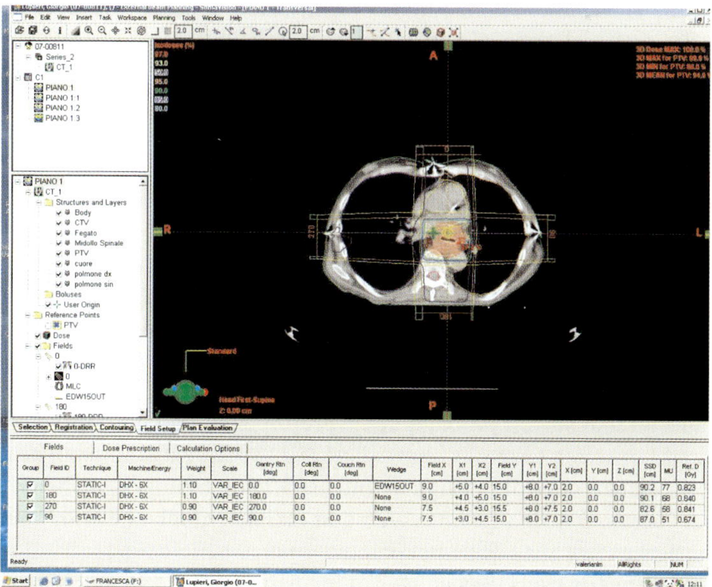

Fig. 5.1 Dose distribution in the axial plane of a CT slice in a case of curative RT and CHT for esophageal cancer

Irradiation of the pericardium or myocardium can produce acute or chronic pericarditis and interstitial fibrosis, correlated with the irradiated volume and dose. Doses to the spinal cord are set under 45 Gy. Irradiation of the lungs can induce radiation pneumonitis and pulmonary fibrosis.

Risk factors for radiation pneumonitis are total dose and treated volume. Radiation pneumonia is observed in a small percentage of patients within 120 days from the end of therapy. Symptoms are fever and cough responding to steroids. Late pulmonary damage is represented by radiation fibrosis; it is observed several months, or years, after the completion of radiotherapy.

Radiotherapy in Cancer of the Stomach

Surgery is also the treatment of choice in gastric cancer. In Western countries diagnosis of the disease is unfortunately late (T2 or more and N+). In cases of full thickness invasion and/or with lymph node involvement, recurrences occur in about 50% of patients within 2 years from surgery. In order to improve local control and survival, many studies have been conducted on multidisciplinary approaches in recent years.

Numerous studies involving CHT alone, both in neoadjuvant and adjuvant regimes failed to produce benefits; in fact in some series, the survival rate in patients submitted to adjuvant CHT worsened. Even RT, when used alone, proved ineffective.

RT alone has been used in the adjuvant phase, producing an increase in local control, without benefits in terms of survival. RT has also been used in the neoadjuvant phase and during surgery with an intraoperative (IORT) method, also with an increase in local control without any advantage in survival.

Currently, the therapeutic standard in locally advanced gastric carcinoma is the concomitant association of adjuvant radiochemotherapy and, in selected cases, neoadjuvant therapy. The main reason for this derives from a randomized phase III study, in which patients with wall invasion and/or lymph node involvement with elevated grading underwent either surgery alone or surgery followed by concomitant radiochemotherapy with 5-FU administered according to the Mayo scheme [9]. The study, in which 556 patients were recruited, showed a statistically significant advantage in terms of 3-year survival and relapse-free survival rate of 50% against 41%, and 48% against 31% for patients treated with a multidisciplinary approach compared to those who underwent surgery alone.

Beyond the issue of local control, the elevated incidence of distant metastasis remains an unresolved problem and therefore another cooperative study, the Cancer and Leukemia Group B Study (CALGB -80101) attempted to produce an increase in distant control through an intensification of adjuvant chemotherapy. The results showed a significant increase in toxicity, combined with a reduction in the appearance of metastasis but without evident benefits in terms of survival.

As with other districts, advantages of the neoadjuvant schedule would derive from greater compliance and radiosensitivity and the absence of delay due to postoperative complications.

Only a few studies with small patient populations have taken this approach, but the available data seem to confirm a better tolerance. Thanks to the downstaging induced by the combined treatment further advantages of the preoperative treatment would be, an increase in surgical resecability and the avoidance intraoperative seeding.

Like other districts, higher radiosensibility is due to a better oxygenation of the tumoral cells. In 1998 Zang published the results of a phase III study with 370 patients affected by carcinoma of the cardias, randomized into 2 groups: the first underwent RT with 40 Gy in 20 fractions in 4 weeks, followed by surgery while the second underwent surgery alone. Local control was 61% in the preoperative group vs. 48% in the other; the data were statistically significant (p <0.05) [10].

A more recent study on the role of the combined preoperative treatment consisting of 33 patients affected by resectable carcinoma of the stomach was published by Ajani et al. At the end of treatment, involving 45 Gy administered in 25 sessions of 1.8 Gy per day, combined with continuous infusion of 5-FU, 58% of patients underwent surgery with an R0 incidence of 70% and T0 30% (no residual tumor). The median survival was 33.7 months with a significant statistical difference between the pT0 cases (63.9 months) and the others (12.6 months) [11].

Based on the knowledge that in patients in pathologic stage T2b and/or N+ the incidence of locoregional recurrence is around 50% and that real extension of the disease during surgical procedures can cause an elevated percentage of incomplete (R+) resections, many investigators have proposed a local intensification of radiation through the employment of intraoperative radiotherapy.

The doses vary between 10 and 18 Gy, based on the extension of the disease, the degree of lymph node involvement, the presence of macroscopic residual tumor and in proximity with critical organs. The advantage of IORT consists of the displacement of the OAR (liver, kidneys, small bowel) from the field and therefore a reduction in toxicity [12].

IORT is carried out on the tumor bed with the area centered on the tripod after completion of tumor removal and prior to surgical reconstruction. The equivalent dose of a single fraction of 20 Gy is very high, being comparable to a dose of 40–45 Gy distributed with conventional fractioning. Abe reported results of a series of 40 patients treated with IORT between 1974 and 1988, showing an increase in locoregional control for patients in advanced stage with aggressive grading [13].

Technical Notes on Radiotherapy

Radiotherapy with external beams is done with conformal 3D technique. The patient is positioned supine in a personalized immobilization device (Wing Board, T Bar) and simulation CT is carried out from the chest to the pelvis after the introduction of oral contrast media. Maximal CT slice thickness should be less than 5 mm. The whole chest and the abdominal cavity are included in the scan; the volumes to be treated are personalized in accordance with the location of the primary tumor. Dose distribution to target and OAR must be evaluated in order to respect tolerance constraints (Fig. 5.2).

The majority of organs present in the upper abdomen may develop acute or late toxicity according to total dose and dose/volume ratio. However, thanks to the employment of multiple personalized filtered fields, doses between 45 and 50.4 Gy in 25–28 sessions of 1.8–2 Gy can be delivered safely.

The employment of CT and PET images to better evaluate the extension of the disease is still investigational; nevertheless, this method appears of particular interest in cases of preoperative treatment in which only the clinical stage is available.

Gastric tumors have a high probability of involving lymph nodes of the greater and lesser curvature, starting from those closest to the origin of the neoplasm (1st level).

The stomach is anatomically divided in 4 parts:

Gastroesophageal junction: In this case the volumes include the medial portion of the left diaphragm and part of the body of the pancreas. If the tumor is staged T4 then the areas need to be widened to include the drain stations of the organs involved. The locoregional lymph node stations are the periesophageal, lower mediastinal, perigastric and tripod [14].

Cardias and fundus: In this case the volumes always include the medial portion of the left diaphragm, the body and ± the tail of the pancreas. The involved lymph node stations are the periesophageal, the pancreaticoduodenal, the perigastric, tripod and splenic hilum.

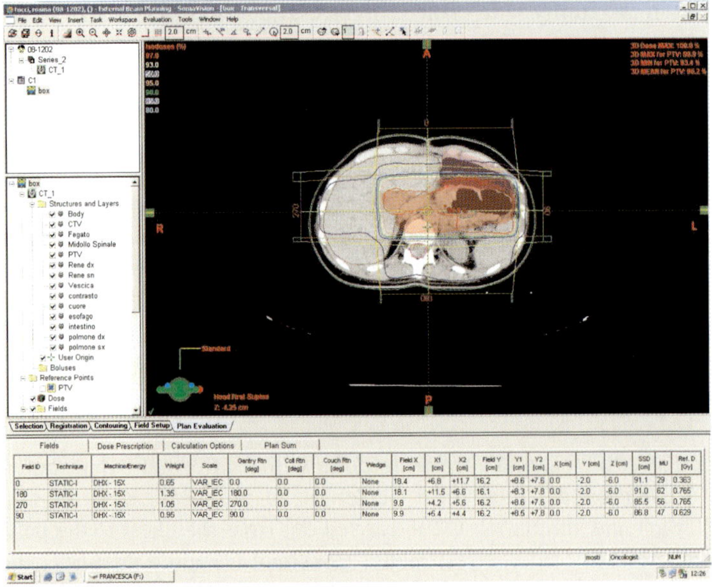

Fig. 5.2 Dose distribution in the axial plane of a CT slice in a case of concomitant adjuvant CHT and RT for cancer of the body of the stomach

Body: The volumes include the body and ± the tail of the pancreas, perigastric, tripod, pancreaticoduodenal and splenic and liver hilum.

Antrum and pylorus: The volumes include the head and the body of the pancreas, the 1st and 2nd parts of the duodenum, perigastric, pancreaticoduodenal, tripod and liver hilum.

The OAR include the possible residual portion of the stomach, liver, kidneys, the spinal cord, the heart and the small bowel. The maximal tolerated dose by the kidneys is 30 Gy on 50% of the volume; normally the most affected kidney is the left one. In order to reduce radiation toxicity, prior evaluation of renal function and total renal volume needs to be evaluated [15].

The most frequent treatment plan uses 4 fields and dose calculation and distribution is performed with a conformal 3D technique. The use of traditional simulator and 2D dose calculation is no longer tolerated.

The use of more complex systems of calculation like IMRT with non conventional non coplanar fields allows a further optimization of dose distribution and better tolerance [16].

Radiotherapy in Cancer of the Pancreas

The prognosis for cancer of the pancreas is very unfavorable due to late diagnosis and elevated incidence of distant metastases at diagnosis. Currently the most used form of radiotherapy in adenocarcinoma of the pancreas is in the adjuvant phase, in association with chemotherapy, after surgical resection.

Radical surgery is the treatment of choice but is only possible in a limited percentage of cases. The frequency of local recurrence varies between 50 and 80% after total macroscopic removal, due to rare microscopically free margins; carcinoma of the pancreas frequently infiltrates the retropancreatic fat, invades the portal vein and the superior mesenteric artery, the lymphovascular and perineural space, and most frequently spreads to the peritoneal cavity and liver. In this setting adjuvant radiotherapy finds a strong rationale and its use becomes even more relevant in cases of residual disease (R+).

The first randomized study in which the effectiveness of an adjuvant treatment was shown was published in 1974 by the GITSG. In that series patients treated with surgery alone were compared to patients in whom surgery was followed by concomitant 5-FU based radiochemotherapy. The results showed efficacy of the combined treatment (median survival 20 months vs. 11 months, 2-year survival rate 45% vs. 15%) [17]. Many other investigators confirmed these results [18].

In order to increase the efficacy of such treatments and to evaluate the possible activity of other molecules, other drugs have been associated with 5-FU; mitomycin C, folic acid and dipiramidol. The best results were obtained associating interferon α to 5-FU: the Virginia Mason Medical Center presented a study with 33 patients, 17 treated with chemotherapy associated with interferon and 16 with the same regimen proposed by GITSG. Results showed a 24-month median survival vs. 18.5 and a 2-year survival rate of 84% vs. 54%. These data were statistically significant (p <0.05). Nevertheless this series showed a significant increase in gastrointestinal grade III/IV toxicity: nausea, vomiting, mucositis and diarrhea [19].

A recent study published in 2003 randomized 34 patients affected by locally advanced pancreatic cancer with 2 possible therapeutic options: 3D conformal radiotherapy associated with concomitant continuous infusion of 5-FU vs. RT in association with weekly gemcitabine. All patients successively underwent maintenance chemotherapy with gemcitabine until progression. The study reported an increase in median survival (6.7 vs. 14.5 months) and response (12% vs. 50%) in the group treated with gemcitabine as well as for pain control (39% vs. 6%), performance status and quality of life [20].

The ESPAC 1 study reported contradictory results; this series was made up of 3 phase III randomized arms: hypofractionated radiotherapy (3 Gy x 10) in association with concomitant 5-FU at a dose of 200 mg/m^2, chemotherapy alone with 5-FU and folic acid and concomitant radiochemotherapy as in the first group, followed by maintenance chemotherapy as in the second group. In this study 285 patients were enrolled and it showed an advantage in terms of survival for patients treated with CHT alone vs. radiochemotherapy of 40 % vs. 30% at 2 years and 21% vs. 8% at 5 years. These data, however, were criticized due to inadequacy of radiation both in terms of dose and fractionation; one more limitation of this study was the absence of restaging after surgery, prior to adjuvant therapy [21].

Another randomized trial – RTOG 9704 – consisted of 442 patients randomized in 2 arms: the first was treated with one course of 5-FU at a dose of 250 mg/m^2 in continuous infusion, while the second was treated with one course of Gemcitabine at a dose of 1000 mg/m^2 [22].

Successively both arms underwent the same concomitant radiochemotherapy at a dose of 50.4 Gy in 28 fractions and 5-FU in continuous infusion at the dose of 200 mg/m^2 for 5 weeks and then two more courses of CHT, consisting of the same schedules subministered prior to radiation: 5-FU in the first arm and Gemcitabine in the second.

Therefore, CHT was carried out for a total of 3 courses: one before radiochemotherapy and 2 after. The median survival was 16.7 months in the 5-FU arm and 18.8 months in the gemcitabine arm with a 3 year survival rate of 21% and 31%, respectively. These data demonstrated the superiority of gemcitabine over 5-FU as an adjuvant treatment when associated with concomitant radiochemotherapy.

Other studies have evaluated the role of the preoperative setting. In fact, advances in diagnostic imaging enable a better evaluation of the real extension of disease without surgical staging, while interventional radiology and endoscopy are able to treat obstructive jaundice with noninvasive methods. This has led many investigators mainly in North America to study the feasibility of a neoadjuvant approach with the purpose of improving local control and eventually increase the incidence of radical surgical procedures thanks to possible downstaging.

The theoretical advantages are notable, and include avoiding delay in the administration of a multimodal treatment and increasing the number of patients who can take advantage of the combined treatment. In fact, because of the postoperative setting, around 25% of cases cannot be submitted to adjuvant therapy and another 1/3 start more than 10 weeks after surgery. Furthermore, preoperative therapy selects patients with better prognosis avoiding surgery in patients who show disseminated disease at the time of restaging. Increasing the percentage of radical procedures thanks to downstaging, providing an increase in radiosensibility and better distribution of drugs thanks to integrity of structures and reducing the risk of intraoperative seeding are further advantages of the technique.

The drugs used are the same as those in adjuvant therapy, such as 5-FU, mitomycin C and gemcitabine, while radiation is delivered with conventional fractionation (45-50, 4 Gy with daily fractions of 1.8 Gy) or hypofractionation (30 Gy in 10 fractions of 3 Gy), eventual IORT, with early results showing a reduction in local recurrences of 10–20% and an increase in radical surgical procedures of 8–16%.

In 1997 Spitz published a series of 142 nonrandomized patients treated with neoadjuvant chemoradiotherapy vs. adjuvant chemoradiation. Both arms used 5-FU. The incidence of toxicity and survival were similar for the 2 groups. The incidence of recurrence was 10% in the preoperative arm and 21% in the adjuvant arm. Furthermore, radiotherapy was not uniform, since patients treated in the neoadjuvant setting received either 30 Gy in 10 fractions or 50.4 Gy in 28 while cases submitted to adjuvant therapy were homogeneously treated with the latter scheme [23].

A more recent study by Hoffmann of the ECOG included 53 patients submitted to neoadjuvant radiochemotherapy consisting of 50.4 Gy in 28 fractions in association with mitomycin C at a dose of 10 mg/m^2 on day 1 and 5-FU at a dose of 1000 mg/m^2 in continuous infusion from days 2 to 5 and from days 29 to 32. After completion of treatment only 41 patients were eligible for surgery. Of these, 17 were not operated because of local or distant progression. Thus, only 24 patients underwent surgery; median survival was 15.7 months and the median follow up 52 months [24]. In conclusion, currently there are no available data showing a real superiority of the neoadjuvant approach.

Preoperative radiotherapy by itself or in association with chemotherapy has been proposed for the treatment of locally advanced disease with the purpose of increasing the percentage of radical interventions with negative borders (R0). Some results would seem to confirm this hypothesis, although the lack of randomized studies does not allow the optimal therapeutic paradigm to be established. Chemoradiotherapy is the only treatment for inoperable neoplasms, even though the 2-year survival is around 10–20%. This affirmation is supported by some randomized and nonrandomized studies that compared radiotherapy alone with combined treatment.

Among these the GITSG study showed an advantage in survival for patients treated with concomitant radiochemotherapy in comparison to cases treated with radiotherapy alone, with a median survival of 42.2 weeks for patients treated with combined therapy and 22.9 weeks for patients treated with radiotherapy alone [25]. In this randomized study 5-FU was administered weekly in bolus and radiotherapy administered with a "split course scheme" that is currently no longer in use. Furthermore, 5-FU in association with radiotherapy is currently administered in continuous infusion. On the basis of this, the guidelines of the National Comprehensive Cancer Network (NCCN) suggest the use of doses of radiations in the order of 50-60 Gy associated with concomitant 5-FU in continuous infusion for inoperable patients with cancer of the pancreas.

More recent studies have been evaluating the use of new molecules to associate with or to replace 5-FU; the most frequently used is Gemcitabine, given its great efficacy in metastatic disease and because of its powerful radio-enhancing action [26].

One of the most recent randomized studies, published in 2003, evaluated 34 patients submitted to 3D conformal radiotherapy, comparing 5-FU in continuous infusion vs. weekly gemcitabine. After the term of concomitant treatment all patients underwent maintenance chemotherapy with gemcitabine up to progression. The results of this study showed an increase in median survival from 6.7 to 14.5 months for patients treated with gemcitabine in comparison with the control group. The percentage of response was also far better in the Gemcitabine group (50% vs. 12%), as well as pain control (39% vs. 6%), performance status and adjusted quality of life [27].

On the other hand, other studies have reported an increase in acute toxicity for patients treated with concomitant gemcitabine without significant difference regarding survival (11 vs. 9, $p = 0.19$) and rate of operable patients (5 of 53 in the Gem group vs. 1 of 61 in the 5-FU group). The efficacy of gemcitabine was also evaluated in association with other molecules with the purpose of dose intensification. In 2007 a study of radiotherapy associated with gemcitabine and cisplatin was published and showed a good tolerance of the intensified regimen in the absence of significant advantages in terms of survival and local control. Recent data would show an advantage of a sequential scheme founded on the rationale of selecting patients in accordance with their response after one or two courses of chemotherapy alone, restaging and eventual association of RT and CHT. IORT is also used in the treatment of cancer of the pancreas. The rationale of IORT is to obtain local dose intensification, without increasing toxicity thanks to the surgical removal of the OAR. In fact, one characteristic of pancreatic neoplasms is the likelihood of diffusion to the liver and peritoneum. IORT is performed in association with external beam radiotherapy and, according to data reported by some investigators, is able to increase local control to 78–81% at one year. Nevertheless, the increase in local control is not associated with a benefit in terms of survival. The administered doses are in the order of 10–20 Gy; in cases of radical surgery doses are around 15 Gy, while in cases of macroscopic residual tumor 18–20 Gy can be reached.

Technical Notes on Radiotherapy

Radiotherapy with external beams is performed using personalized immobilization devices, simulation CT with slice thickness under 5 mm, using 3–4 isocentric, personalized filtered fields, and dose distribution calculated with conformal 3D technique in which the target and the OAR are contoured (Fig. 5.3). The target volume includes the clinically recognizable neoplasm in the case of preoperative or curative treatment or the tumoral bed in the case of adjuvant therapy, the peripancreatic and the paraortic lymph nodes, from a plane including the lower margin of the D11 till the L3–L4 space, the celiac tripod and the mesenteric lymph nodes. Use of PET-CT for the preoperative approach is still investigational. Once the target and the organ at risk are drawn, and the treatment plan has been compiled, it is mandatory to evaluate the dose/volume histograms in order to respect the dose/volume constraints. The RTOG 9704 study has outlined some guidelines for the tolerance of OAR.

Liver and small bowel should be excluded as much as possible from the entry fields. The V30 of the liver should not exceed 60% of the total volume of the organ (percentage of volume included within an equivalent total dose of 30 Gy administered with conventional fractioning). The dose limit for the spinal cord is 40–45 Gy (not depending on volume) and should not be encompassed.

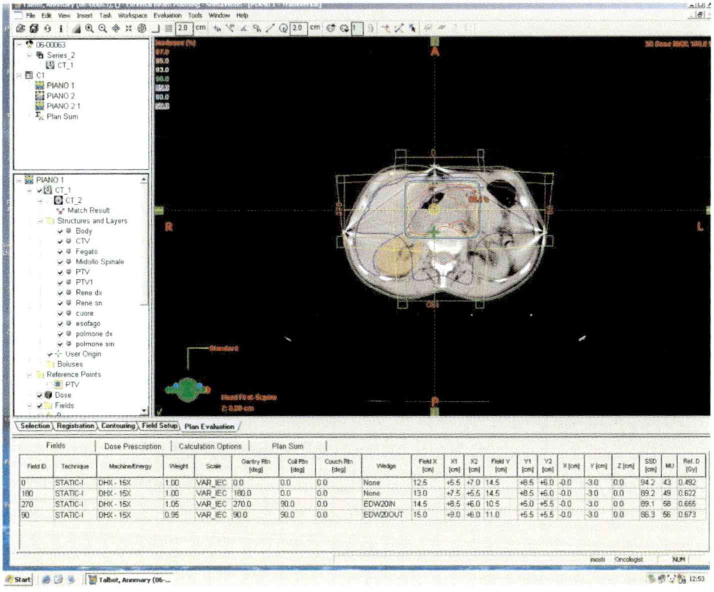

Fig. 5.3 Dose distribution in the axial plane for adjuvant therapy in carcinoma of the head of the pancreas

Particular attention is reserved to the dose absorbed by the kidneys; prior to treatment renal function is evaluated in order to respect dose/volume constraints. The target volume is determined by the primary location of the disease (head, body, tail).

Implementation of IMRT increases dose/volume distribution for target and OAR. In this subset of patients, a limitation in the use of IMRT derives from the increase in duration of each session and from the need for rigorous positioning which can prove difficult in patients with poor performance status [28].

Radiotherapy in Cancer of the Rectum

The principal treatment for resectable carcinoma of the rectum is surgery. Considering that in the locally advanced stage between 20 and 50% of patients suffer recurrence has made adjuvant therapies necessary. Within this interdisciplinary approach radiotherapy plays a fundamental role, regarding survival, incidence of local recurrence, quality of life and organ preservation. Adjuvant radiotherapy, alone or in association with chemotherapy, can be administered preoperatively or postoperatively. The goals of postoperative therapy are to reduce local recurrence and to improve overall survival, whereas preoperative treatment also adds the potential benefit of sphincter preservation. In the 1980s and 1990s data from prospective randomized studies answered many questions on the role of postoperative radiotherapy related to patient selection, the eventual association with chemotherapy and the type of drugs to associate with radiation. Two randomized studies – the GISTG 7175 and the Mayo C/NCCTG – compared surgery alone with surgery plus radiation and chemotherapy [29, 30]. In the first study patients were submitted to pelvic radiation with a dose of 50.4 Gy in 28 fractions of 1.8 Gy and the other group associated pelvic radiation with 6-8 cycles of chemotherapy with 5-FU. On the basis of these results, the 1990 "National Cancer Institute Consensus Conference" established that combined modalities therapy represented the standard of care for patients with T3 and/or positive lymph nodes. Further studies showed that best efficacy, associated with better tolerance, was when radiation was associated with 5-FU in continuous infusion and that combination with other molecules does not determine a significant improvement in results [31].

During the last few years the continuous progress of diagnostic techniques has sensibly reduced the principal limitation of preoperative radiotherapy, i.e. lack of pathologic staging which may lead to over- or undertreatment. On the basis of this evidence studies aimed at evaluating the efficacy of preoperative therapy have been investigated. Exclusive preoperative or neoadjuvant chemoradiation can be administered with two different modalities. The first uses an intensified hypofractionated regimen, and has been mainly used in northern European countries (Sweden, Norway and The Netherlands), consisting of 5 consecutive sessions of 5 Gy for a total dose of 25 Gy. The second method consists of conventional fractioning and doses in the order of 50–55 Gy in 28–33 consecutive sessions. Both approaches are valid in increasing local control; the intensified hypofractionated regimen, thanks also to its statistical power, has been the first to show not only an improvement in local control (12% vs. 27%, p <0.001) but also of survival rate (5-year survival rate 58% vs. 48%, p = 0.004). Further studies confirmed that in stage II and III, the addition of neoadjuvant hypofractionated radiotherapy improved results (local relapse at 2 years 2.4% vs. 8.2%, p <0.001) even in the presence of a certified total mesorectal excision. Disadvantages of this approach are lack of downstaging and eventual suboptimal therapy for N+ cases which may require associated chemotherapy. Furthermore, this regimen is associated with an increase in gastrointestinal toxicity and of sphincter dysfunctions. When considering conventional fractionation, the available data show superiority of associated therapy vs. radiation alone. Two randomized studies are available: the EORTC 22921 and FFCD 9203, which reported a significant increase in complete responses (14% vs. 5% and 10% vs. 3%) not associated with an increase in survival [32]. The available data confirm that preoperative radiotherapy, whether in association with chemotherapy or not, obtains better results than postoperative radiotherapy. The first randomized trial which showed superiority of neoadjuvant radiotherapy compared to adjuvant was the Uppsala Trial, in which neoadjuvant radiotherapy with a dose of 25 Gy in 5 fractions was compared to postoperative radiotherapy with a dose of 60 Gy in 30 fractions. In the preoperative arm there was a significant statistical reduction in local recurrence (13% vs. 22%) without benefit in survival.

More recently, after the failure of the RTOG 94-01 and NSABP R-03 studies due to limited recruitment, a German multicenter randomized trial compared combined preoperative radiochemotherapy at a dose of 50.4 Gy in 28 fractions associated with 5-FU in continuous infusion with the same therapy administered in the adjuvant modality. The preoperative group showed a significant improvement in local control (7% vs. 11%) and, in the low-lying tumors, an increased percentage of sphincter preservation (19% vs. 39%) [33].

Further advantages of downstaging are represented by the improvement of surgical results in terms of negative radial margins and for its prognostic value which influences further therapy. In fact, in patients submitted to preoperative radiotherapy, one of the more important prognostic factors currently recognized is status of radial margins. The possible infiltration of this is associated with an increase of recurrence. Nagtegaal reported different prognostic significance of positive radial margin in patients submitted to preoperative RT and CHT vs. the same findings after surgery alone. Positive radial margins after preoperative therapy are associated with an increase in the incidence of distant metastasis and a reduction in survival [34].

In order to increase organ preservation, neoadjuvant radiotherapy alone or in association with chemotherapy has also been used in the early stage for ultralow-lying tumors. The current trend in this subgroup of patients is to perform a full thickness local excision after neoadjuvant therapy; if the pathologic evaluation of the sample shows complete tumor regression (TRG) 0–2, and therefore a complete response, conventional surgery may be avoided; on the other hand if vital cells persist (TRG 3), radical surgery is recommended. The use of PET to evaluate response to therapy is still under investigation [35–37]. Currently, cancer of the rectum is diagnosed in the majority of cases when still technically operable. But in some cases, extension of the disease does not consent radical surgical procedures. In the absence of distant metastases, combined chemoradiotherapy is advisable with the objective of obtaining a downstaging that will allow radical surgery.

IORT has precise indications also for extraperitoneal rectal cancer. It should be used in association with external beam radiation as a local dose intensifier on the surgical bed with doses in the order of 10–15 Gy after radical resection or 12–18 Gy in cases of macroscopic residual tumor. Doses above 18 Gy determine a significant increase in late neuropathy. IORT guarantees an increase in local control, but no increase in survival has been reported so far. In cases of systemic dissemination, radiation has a palliative finality. In this case, volumes are reduced. The standard dose is 30 Gy in 10 sessions of 3 Gy; around 50% of patients show a significant reduction of at least one symptom.

Treatment of recurrences is complex because of its heterogeneity (local recurrence alone, local disease associated with distant metastases, level of infiltration of pelvic walls) and because of possible previous treatment. Suzuki classified pelvic recurrences according to wall infiltration: from F0 (no pelvic wall infiltration) to F4 (all 4 pelvic walls involved) [38]. A multicenter study published by the Sacred Heart Catholic University of Rome reported results of a series of 47 patients affected by local recurrent rectal cancer. All patients underwent RT with 45 Gy, associated with continuous infusion of 5-FU (225 mg/m^2) and IORT at a dose of 10–15 Gy; 5-year survival was 21% with a 22% relapse-free survival. The same investigators reported an experience of re-irradiation with multiple fractioning, (1.2 Gy, BID) at a dose of 30 Gy on the pelvis, with overdose up to 40.2 Gy on recurrent disease associated with concomitant continuous 5-FU infusion at a dose of 225 mg/m^2. Results, with a median follow up of 36 months, were a median survival of 42 months and a 48% median relapse-free survival [39].

Technical Notes on Radiotherapy

The volumes extend from the L5–S1 space up to the ischium, using 3D conformal technique with multiple personalized fields. The canalis sacralis is included. The external iliac nodes are inserted in the case of positive lymph nodes. The inguinal lymph nodes are included in the case of involvement of the anal canal. In cases of abdominal-perineal amputation the perineum is also included.

Doses vary from 25 Gy in 5 fractions to 60 Gy in 30–33 sessions of 1.8–2 Gy. Doses in the preoperative setting are generally lower (40–45 Gy on the pelvis plus 5–10 Gy on the tumor), or 25 Gy in 5 fractions of 5 Gy, while in the adjuvant treatment doses vary from 50 to 60 Gy (45–50 Gy on the pelvis and overdose of 10–15 Gy on the tumor bed). Patients are positioned prone, using personalized immobilization devices which displace the small bowel from portals (Belly Board, Up Down Table). Simulation CT is performed to identify target and OAR (small bowel, femurs, bladder and gonads) (Fig. 5.4). Also for rectal cancer, the use of IMRT allows dose intensification with no increase in toxicity. PET imaging is still investigational to better define the real extension of the disease.

For intraoperative treatment, electrons with energy between 6 and 10 Mev are used, aimed at the surgical bed after removal of the neoplasm and before reconstruction. Doses are in the order of 10–15 Gy. In determining the area a margin of 2 cm around the initial extension of the disease is considered adequate. In cases of residual disease, delivered doses are slightly higher but doses and volumes should be limited to avoid toxicity to the urethers, sacrum and bladder.

Radiotherapy in Cancer of the Anal Canal

Concomitant radiochemotherapy is currently the standard of care for treatment of carcinoma of the anal canal. In the past most patients were submitted to radical surgery with abdominal-perineal amputation. The consequent morbidity to such treatment was high and surgery was followed by an elevated incidence of recurrences [40]. Currently radiochemotherapy is considered the first therapeutic option when pretreatment staging confirms a disease at least T2 or N+ while in some cases of T1 N0 the option for an exclusive local excision can be consid-

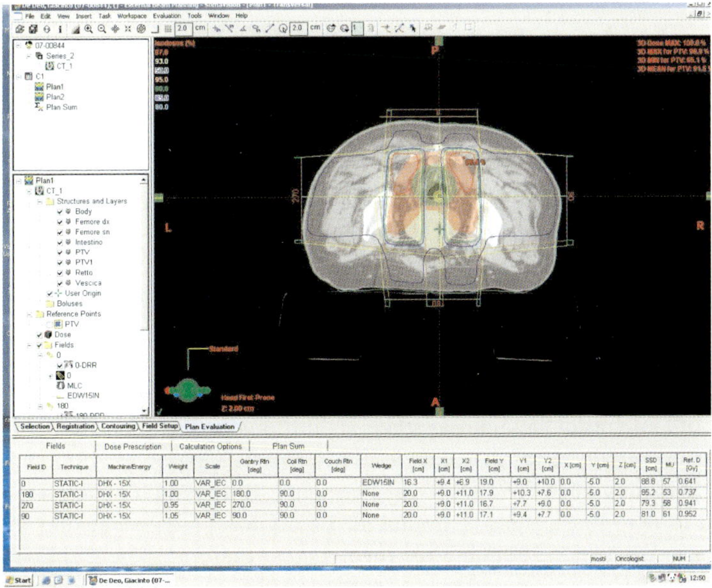

Fig. 5.4 Dose distribution in the axial plane in a case of neoadjuvant chemoradiation therapy for rectal cancer

ered. Nigro was the first to publish a series reporting an elevated incidence of complete remission after concomitant radiochemotherapy with 5-FU, mitomycin C and external beam radiation [41].

Even in the absence of perspective randomized studies comparing radiochemotherapy and surgery, the advantages of the conservative option are so evident, both in terms of efficacy and quality of life, that the surgical option has been dismissed. The literature reports an incidence of complete remission of around 2/3 of patients at the end of therapy; this value varies between 85% for cases in stage I–II and 50% for those in stage III.

The drugs used are 5-FU in continuous infusion during the whole period of the RT or administered during the 1st and 5th week of RT (the doses are in the order of 200–250 mg/m^2 in continuous infusion or 1000 mg/m^2 in the weekly bases). 5-FU is associated either with mitomycin C or cisplatin in bolus on the 1st and the 29th day at doses respectively of 10 or 70–100 mg/m^2 [42]. Efficacy of 5-FU associated with mitomycin or cisplatin was evaluated in the randomized RTOG 98-11 trial [43]. The results of this study showed similarities between both schedules in terms of overall and local survival, while they showed a higher incidence of colostomies in the cisplatin group. Another phase II study denominated RTOG 92-08 tested efficacy of a "split course" of two weeks during chemoradiation with the purpose of reducing acute toxicity. The results showed a higher incidence of recurrence in patients submitted to the split course than in the control group, therefore, the current recommendation is to perform chemoradiation continuously [44].

Technical Notes on Radiotherapy

In the initial stages (T1–2, N0) delivered doses are in the order of 36 Gy on the pelvis and 40–45 Gy on the initial tumor. In more advanced stages ($\geq$ T3 $\pm$ N+) doses are in the order of 40–45 Gy on the pelvis and of 59–64 Gy on the tumor (Fig. 5.5). The boost can be carried out with external X-rays or electrons, dedicated endocavitary applicators or with brachitherapy. Patients are normally positioned supine with the purpose of reducing inhomogeneity of the natural curves of the pelvis and the perineum. The upper limit of the fields are set at the level of the bifurcation of the common iliac arteries, while the lateral margin has to include the inguinal lymph node stations. The lower limit is set caudally to the anus delimited with a radiopaque marker. Normally the patient is set in a personalized immobilization device and some institutions prefer to position the patient prone, using small bowel dislocators (Belly Board, Up down table) and adding a bolus to homogenize the dose to the perineum. If no lymph nodes are affected, the total dose to these areas is around 30–36 Gy for T1–T2 stage and 45 Gy for T3-4 stage. In cases of lymph node involvement these areas are surdosed up to 50–60 Gy. The acute side effects of treatment are enteroproctitis and inguinal and perineal dermatitis which can lead to the temporary suspension of treatment. Hematologic toxicity is rare with an incidence of Grade 3 around 2%.

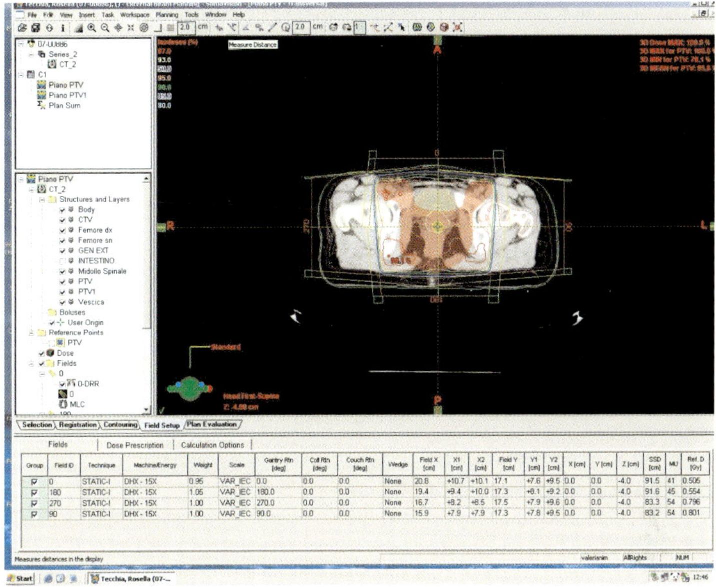

Fig. 5.5 Dose distribution in the axial plane in a case of curative concomitant RT and CHT for carcinoma of the anal canal

Functionality of the sphincter after treatment depends more on the degree of initial involvement than on possible radiation damage. Considering the high efficacy of curative radiochemotherapy even in advanced stages, currently around one third of these patients develop distant metastasis without local recurrence. Unfortunately distant disease is relatively resistant to systemic chemotherapy and complete remission for metastatic disease is of anecdotal relevance.

References

1. Herskovich AMK, al-Sarraf M, Leichman L (1992) Combined chemotherapy and radiotherapy compared with radiotherapy alone in patients with cancer of esophagus. N Engl J Med 326:1593–1598
2. Minsky BD (2006) Primary combined-modality therapy for esophageal cancer. Oncology (Williston Park) 20(5):497–505
3. Zhao KL, Wang Y, Shi XH (2003) Late course accelerated hyperfractionated radiotherapy for clinical T1-2 esophageal carcinoma. World J Gastroenterol 9:1374–1376
4. Urba SG, Porringer MB,Turrisi A (2001) Randomized trial of pre-operative chemoradiation vs. surgery alone in patients with locoregional esophageal carcinoma. J Clin Oncol 19:305–313
5. Bosset JF, Gignoux M, Triboulet JP et al (1997) Chemoradiotherapy followed by surgery compared with surgery alone in squamous-cell cancer of esophagus. N Engl J Med 337:161–167
6. Walsh TN, Noonan N, Hollywood D (1996) Comparison of multimodal therapy and surgery for esophageal carcinoma. N Engl J Med 335:462–467

7. Bonnetain F, Bouche O, Michel P (2006) A comparative longitudinal quality of life study using the Spitzer quality of life index in a randomized multicenter phase III trial (FFCD 91029) Ann Oncol 17:827–834

8. Harvey JC, Fleishman EH, Bellotti JE (1993) Intracavitary radiation in the treatment of advanced esophageal carcinoma: a comparison of high dose rate vs. low dose rate brachitherapy. J Surg Oncol 52:101–104

9. Macdonald JS, Smalley SR, Benedetti J et al (2001) Chemoradiotherapy after surgery compared with surgery alone for adenocarcinoma of the stomach or gastroesophageal junction. N Engl J Med 345:725

10. Zhang ZX, Gu XZ, Yin WB et al (1999) Ramdomized clinical trial on the combination of preoperative irradiation and surgery in the treatment of adenocarcinoma of gastric cardia (AGC). Report on 370 patients. Int J Radiat Oncol Biol Phys 44(5):1185

11. Ajani JA, Mansfield PF, Janjan N et al (2004) Multi-institutional trial of preoperative chemoradiotherapy in patients with potentially respectable gastric carcinoma. J Clin Oncol 22:2774–2780

12. Gunderson L, Tepper J (2007) Clinical radiation oncology, 2nd edn. Churchill Livingstone Elsevier, Philadelphia

13. Abe M, Takahashi M, Ono K (1988) Japan gastric trials on intraoperative radiation therapy. Int J Radiat Oncol Biol Phys 15(6):1431–1433

14. Smalley SS, Gunderson L, Tepper J et al (2002) Gastric surgical adjuvant radiotherapy consensus report. Rationale and treatment implementation. Int J Radiat Oncol Biol Phys 52:282

15. Pemberton L, Coote J, Perry V et al (2006) Adjuvant chemoradiotherapy for gastric carcinoma: dosimetric implications of conventional gastric bed irradiation and toxicity. Clinical Oncology 18:663–668

16. Soyfer V, Corn BW, Melamud A et al (2007) Three-dimensional non-coplanar conformal radiotherapy yields better results than traditional beam arrangements for adjuvant treatment of gastric cancer. Int J Radiat Oncol Biol Phys 2:364–369

17. Gastrointestinal Tumor Study Group (1987) Further evidence of effective adjuvant combined radiation and chemotherapy following curative resection of pancreatic cancer. Cancer 59:2006–2010

18. Sohn TA, Yeo CJ, Cameron JL (2000) Resected adenocarcinoma of the pancreas – 616 patients: results, outcomes, and prognostic indicators. J Gastrointest Surg 4(6):567–579

19. Regine WF, Winter KW, Abrams R et al (2006) RTOG 9704 a phase III study of adjuvant pre and post chemoradiation (CRT) 5-FU vs. gemcitabine (G) for resected pancreatic adenocarcinoma. J Clin Oncol 24(Suppl 18):A–4007, 180s

20. Haddock MG, Swaminathan R, Foster NR et al (2007) Gemcitabine, cisplatin and radiotherapy for patients with locally advanced pancreatic adenocarcinoma: results of the North Central Cancer Treatment Group Phase II Study N9942. J Clin Oncol 25:2567–2572

21. Morris SL, Beaslye M, Leslie M et al (2004) Chemotherapy for pancreatic cancer. N Engl J Med 350:2713

22. Regine WF, Winter KW, Abrams R et al (2006) RTOG 9704, a phase III study of adjuvant pre- and post-chemoradiation (CRS) 5-FU vs. gemcitabine (G) for resected pancreatic adenocarcinoma. J Clin Oncol 185:4007

23. Spitz FR, Abbruzzese JL, Lee JL (1997) Preoperative and postoperative chemoradiation strategies in patients treated with pancreaticoduodenectomy for adenocarcinoma of the pancreas. J Clin Oncol 15(3):928–937

24. Hoffmann JP, Cooper HS, Nancy A (1998) Preoperative chemoterapy of chemoradiotherapy of treatment of adenocarcinoma of the pancreas and ampulla of Vater. J Hepatobil Pancr Surg 5:251–252

25. Moertel CG, Frytak S, Hahn RG (1981) Therapy of locally unresectable pancreatic carcinoma: a randomized comparison of high dose radiation alone, moderate dose radiation and high dose radiation + 5-fluorouracil. The Gastrointestinal Tumor Study Group. Cancer 48:1705–1710

26. Oettle H, Neuhaus P (2007) Adjuvant therapy in pancreatic cancer: a critical appraisal.

Drugs 67(16):2293–2310

27. Li CP, Chao Y, Chi KH et al (2003) Concurrent chemoradiotherapy treatment of locally advanced pancreatic cancer: gemcitabine vs. 5-fluorouracil, a randomized controlled study. Int J Radiat Oncol Biol Phys 57(1):98–104

28. Milano MT, Chmura SJ, Garafalo MC (2004) Intensity-modulated radiotherapy in treatment of pancreatic and bile duct malignancies: toxicity and clinical outcome. Int J Radiat Oncol Biol Phys 59:445

29. Gastrointestinal Tumor Study Group (1984) Adjuvant therapy of colon cancer. Results of a prospectively randomized trial. N Engl J Med 312:1465

30. O'Connel MJ, Martenson JA, Wiland HS et al (1994) Improving adjuvant therapy for rectal cancer by combining protected infusion fluorouracil with radiation therapy after curative surgery. N Engl J Med 331:502–507

31. O'Connell MJ (2002) Improving adjuvant therapy in stage II and III rectal cancer to define the optimal sequence of chemotherapy and radiotherapy: a preliminary report. J Clin Oncol 20:1751–1758

32. Bosset JF (2004) Does the addition of chemotherapy to preoperative radiotherapy increase the pathological response in patients with resected rectal cancer? Proc ASCO 22:247

33. Sauer R, Becker H, Homenberger W et al (2004) Preoperative chemoradiotherapy as compared with postoperative chemoradiotherapy for locally advanced rectal cancer. New Engl J Med 351:11–20

34. Nagtegaal ID, Quirke P (2008) What is the role for the circumferential margin in the modern treatment of rectal cancer? J Clin Oncol 26(2):303–312

35. Roedel C (2004) Tumor regression grade as a prognostic factor in patients with locally advanced rectal cancer treated with preoperative radiochemotherapy. Int J Radiat Oncol Biol Phis 60(1):S140

36. Bonnen M, Crane C, Vauthey JN et al (2004) Long term results using local excision after preoperative chemoradiation among selected T3 rectal cancer patients. Int J Radiat Oncol Biol Phys 60(4):1098–1105

37. Larson SM, Schoder H, Yeung H (2004) Positron emission tomography / computerized tomography functional imaging of esophageal and colorectal cancer. Cancer J 10:243–250

38. Suzuki K, Dozois RR, Devine RM (1996) Curative reoperations for locally recurrent rectal cancer. Dis Colon Rectum 39(7):730–736

39. Valentini V, Morganti AG, De Franco A (1999) Chemoradiation with or without intraoperative radiation therapy in patients with locally recurrence of rectal carcinoma: prognostic factors and long term outcome. Cancer 86(12):2612–2624

40. Ryan DP, Compton CC, Mayer RJ (2000) Carcinoma of the anal canal. N Engl J Med 342:792–800

41. Nigro ND, Seydal HG, Considine B et al (1983) Combined preoperative radiation and chemotherapy for squamous-cell carcinoma of the anal canal. Cancer 51(10):1826–1829

42. Crehange G, Bosset M, Lorchel F et al (2006) Combining cisplatin and Mitomycin with radiotherapy in anal carcinoma. Dis Colon Rectum 50:43–49

43. Ajani JA, Winter KA, Gunderson LL et al (2006) Intergroup RTOG 98-11: a phase III randomized study of 5-fluorouracil (5-FU), mitomycin, and radiotherapy vs. 5-FU cisplatin and radiotherapy in carcinoma of the anal canal. J Clin Oncol 24: 18S, abstract 4009

44. Konski AA, Winter K, John M et al (2007) Evaluation of planned treatment breaks during radiation therapy for anal cancer: update of Radiation Therapy Oncology Group (RTOG) 92-08. J Clin Oncol Gastrointestinal Cancers Symposium. Abstract 297

Part 2
Personal Experiences and Selected Series

Chapter 6

Surgical Treatment of Colorectal Metastases to the Liver

Genoveffa Balducci, Paolo Mercantini, Niccolò Petrucciani,
Vincenzo Ziparo

Introduction

The liver is the most common site of metastasis from colorectal cancer: about
50% of patients affected by colorectal cancer develop liver metastases during the
course of their disease [1]; of these, 25% present with synchronous liver metastases, whereas an additional 25% develop metachronous hepatic metastases.
Approximately 148,800 cases of colorectal cancer are estimated for 2008 in the
United States, with more than 60,000 cases of liver metastases [2]. Patients with
untreated metastatic colorectal cancer have a poor prognosis with a median survival of 6 to 12 months [3]. Surgical therapy for colorectal liver metastases
remains the only potentially curative treatment. Despite recent advances in systemic chemotherapy, the median survival for unresected patients ranges from 12
to 24 months with uncommon long-term survival, while the 5-year survival rate
after surgery ranges from 25 to 58%. These results are expected to improve with
better patient selection and multimodal approaches. Therefore, when indicated,
resection of colorectal metastases to the liver should always be considered.

In this work we report our experience on 93 patients who underwent liver
resection for colorectal metastases at "La Sapienza" University of Rome in the
last twenty years.

Methods

Between 1988 and 2008, 93 consecutive patients with colorectal metastases to
the liver were observed, until 2002at the Department of Surgery "Pietro Valdoni"
and then at Sant'Andrea Hospital, "La Sapienza" University of Rome. The preoperative diagnosis of colorectal liver metastases was based mainly on computed tomography (CT; or, from 1998, spiral CT). A historical series included 74
patients treated from 1988 to 2004; since 2005, a prospective series of 19
patients was enrolled with clinicopathologic and follow-up data for each patient
in a computerized database which was regularly updated for tumor recurrence
and survival status. Indications for surgery in each patient was discussed with

A. Bolognese, L. Izzo (eds.), *Surgery in Multimodal Management of Solid Tumors.*
©Springer-Verlag Italia 2009

the oncologists and other physicians having a role in the treatment of colorectal metastases. In accordance with the literature, we considered patients candidates to surgery whenever we could obtain a curative resection (R0) preserving as much liver parenchyma as possible. Contraindications for resection were: extended liver involvement (>5 segments, 70% invasion, all hepatic veins infiltrated), Child Class B and C cirrhosis, and major cardiovascular or pulmonary contraindications to surgery. Resection was considered "major" if three or more segments were removed, according to Couinaud's classification. Intraoperative ultrasound was routinely performed in all patients to detect tumor invasion into the major branches of the portal or the hepatic veins and the presence of lesions in the contralateral lobe. After resection, we routinely performed histological examination to define the surgical procedures as curative (R0). Hospital mortality was defined as death within 30 days after operation, including operative deaths. Tumor recurrence was considered as evidence of hepatic tumoral lesions after a curative resection. All patients discharged were followed up every 3 months in the first year and every 6 months thereafter. The follow-up consisted of physical examination, blood tests, serological liver function tests, and liver ultrasound or CT scan. The last follow-up evaluation was performed in May 2008.

Results

The first series includes 74 patients, 39 males and 35 females, treated from 1988 to 2004; 38 (51%) were less than 60 years old. In 52 cases (70.3%) the primary tumor was colonic, whereas 22 patients (29.7%) had a rectal neoplasm. According to Dukes classification, 31 patients (41.9%) had stage B and 43 (58.1%) stage C tumors. Liver lesions were synchronous in 20 cases (27%) and metachronous in 54 (73%). In 40 patients only one lobe was involved (54%). In all 74 patients a total of 88 hepatectomies were performed, 61 (69.3%) non anatomical and 27 (30.7%) anatomical, of which 12 were major hepatectomies (13.6%). Operative mortality and morbidity were 2.7 and 19%, respectively. In this series 3-year and 5-year survival were 62 and 39%, respectively.

From 2005 we started a prospective study enrolling all patients submitted to hepatic resection for colorectal metastases. This series includes 19 patients, 9 males and 10 females; six of whom were less than 60 years old at the time of the first colectomy. The primary tumor site was the rectum in 10 cases (52.6%), the left colon in 8 (42.1%) and the right colon in 1 (5.3%). According to Dukes classification, local stage of primary tumor was Dukes A in 2 patients, Dukes B in 1 patient, Dukes C in 16 patients. Ten patients (52.6%) had synchronous metastases. Hepatic metastases were treated 22 times in 19 patients; lesions were unilateral in 14 cases (63.6%) and bilateral in 8 (36.4%). In 8 cases (36.4%) liver lesions were initially considered unresectable; these patients underwent surgery after downstaging of the disease obtained by chemotherapy.

In those 19 patients we performed 22 hepatectomies, 3 patients receiving re-

resection after recurrence. Hepatectomies were anatomical, all major, 4 times (18.2%) and non anatomical, 18 (81.8%). Hepatic resection was considered liver-curative in 86.4% of cases and globally curative in 77.3.% No operative mortality was observed in this series. Complications occurred in 4 cases (18.2%): biliary leak, intestinal occlusion, intestinal perforation and hemorrhage. Mean duration of hospital stay was 16 days.

Four patients died during the follow-up, all with disease. Actuarial survival rate at 30 months is as high as 67%.

Discussion

In the past, patients with liver metastases from colorectal cancer were considered untreatable with surgery, because the hematogenous spread of tumor cells to the liver was thought to indicate the presence of an already systemic disease, not susceptible to local treatment. Furthermore, the high morbidity and mortality traditionally associated with liver surgery did not justify the surgical exeresis of liver metastases. In contrast, data collected over the last thirty years demonstrates that liver metastases from colorectal cancer may actually be the only secondary manifestation of the disease. This concept of "limited metastatic disease" constitutes the physiopathologic rationale behind considering liver resection as the only potentially curative treatment. Improvement of imaging techniques and introduction of new devices (MR angiography, MR-cholangiopancreatography, spiral-CT, PET, PET-CT, intraoperative ultrasonography, explorative laparoscopy and laparoscopic ultrasonography), advances in surgical techniques (selective liver ischemia, hepatic high-energy ultrasonic dissection) and finally the tendency towards selective surgical procedures (segmentectomies, subsegmentectomies, atypical resections), aimed at sparing hepatic healthy tissue, have lowered operative mortality rates in specialized centers to close to 0%, with in-hospital mortality rates lower than 5% and morbidity rates ranging from 20 to 50% [4–15]. The most frequent causes of perioperative mortality are liver failure and bleeding, occurring in 1–5% of major hepatic resections [16–17].

Although there are currently no randomized trials evaluating the efficacy in terms of survival and relapses of surgical treatment compared to other possible therapies (e.g. chemotherapy), many prospective studies have demonstrated that surgery is the only treatment able to increase long-term survival [18]. Currently the median survival for patients with colorectal metastases undergoing hepatectomy ranges from 24 to 74 months; 5-year survival ranges from 23 to 58% and 10-year survival approaches more than 20% [4–15] (Table 6.1). This report concurs with the literature that hepatic resection is a safe and effective therapy, with a mortality rate of 0% in the last three years of our experience and an actuarial overall survival rate of 67% at 30 months for 19 patients treated in the last three years. These data justify the optimism regarding the increasingly aggressive approach being offered to many patients with liver metastases from colorectal cancer. Furthermore, this study demonstrates a favorable trend in decreased mor-

Table 6.1 Short and long-term survival after hepatic resections for colorectal metastases

Author	No.	Perioperative mortality (%)	1 year (%)	5 years (%)	10 years (%)
Schindl et al. [4]	153	–	84	36	–
Wei et al. [5]	423	1.6	93	47	28
Malik et al. [6]	687	3.0	–	45	–
Arru et al. [7]	297	4.0	91	27	17
Ambiru et al. [8]	168	3.5	81	26	–
Nuzzo et al. [9]	185	1.0	–	38	23
Laurent et al. [10]	311	3.0	86	36	–
Viganò et al. [11]	125	3.0	93	23	16
Fong et al. [12]	1001	3.0	89	37	22
Choti et al. [13]	226	1.0	93	40	–
Fernandez et al. [14]	100	1.0	86	58	–
Pawlik et al. [15]	557	1.0	97	58	–

tality rates over time. Unfortunately, only 5–10% of patients with colorectal metastases to the liver are candidates for curative resection.

Multimodal approaches were developed to increase the number of patients undergoing potentially curative surgery. The use of portal vein embolization, inducing hypertrophy of the controlateral liver, can increase the number of candidates for surgery [19]. Chemotherapy agents allow a subset of previously unresectable patients to undergo liver surgery after tumor downstaging: about 15–20% of patients with unresectable disease have significant tumor downstaging and can be candidates for subsequent liver resection with good survival results, as reported by Adam [20]. Radiofrequency ablation can be used combined with hepatic resection in patients who would otherwise be considered unresectable; the main indication for ablation is a subgroup of patients who do not meet the criteria for resectability, but are candidates for liver-directed therapy based on the presence of liver-only disease [21].

The success of surgical treatment is partially linked to an improvement in patient selection that has occurred over the last thirty years. The factors considered are clinical status, extension of liver metastases, type and extension of hepatic resection in order to preserve adequate amount of healthy tissue, and biological features of the tumor. In recent years, many authors have focused their attention on the study of prognostic factors allowing the identification of subgroups of patients who can benefit from surgical treatment. Though many parameters have been proposed, only the prediction of positive resection margins and the presence of extrahepatic disease are strictly correlated to an early develop of relapses and to therapeutic failure. In patients with isolated pulmonary metastases good results can be obtained associating lung resection with hepatectomy [22]; Elias et al. [23] reported a 5-year survival rate of 29% in patients undergoing hepatectomy for colorectal liver metastases and simultaneous resection of extrahepatic disease. Age and sex do not affect short and long-term survival after hepatic resections. A number of other factors were detected, such as lymph node involvement by the primary tumor, a short disease-free interval between the primary tumor and the development of liver metastases, the presence of satellite nodules, a high preoperative CEA level and the extension of the hepatic disease (roughly 50% of the parenchyma). However a unanimous consensus on the impact of each factor on long-term results and relapse conditions has not been reached by the various authors.

On this subject Fong, in a study of 1001 patients, suggested a schematic and streamlined method of patient selection composed of 5 criteria, called the *Clinical Risk Score* (CRS) [12]. The five criteria are:

1. Size of the liver metastases >5 cm
2. Disease-free interval between primary cancer and liver metastases <12 months
3. Number of liver metastases >1
4. Nodal involvement by the primitive tumor
5. Preoperative CEA >200 ng/mL

Each parameter of CRS constitutes a negative prognostic factor, related to a 5-year survival worsening. However, none of these criteria can be considered an absolute contraindication to liver resection. Recently some investigators have suggested that molecular tumor biomarkers, such as Ki-67 labeling index, human telomerase reverse transcriptase expression, tritiated thymidine uptake and thymidylate synthase expression may be useful for predicting survival after resection. However preoperative factors should not be used to exclude patients from surgical consideration, because patients with multiple negative factors can still derive a significant survival benefit from hepatic resection.

Currently the definition of resectability represents a paradigm shift: resectability is no more defined by what is removed, but rather decisions should now focus on what will remain after resection. Therefore hepatic colorectal metastases should be defined resectable when it is anticipated that the disease can be completely resected, two adjacent liver segments can be spared, adequate vascular inflow and outflow and biliary drainage can be preserved and the volume of the liver remaining after resection will be adequate [18]. In general 20% of the total liver volume appears to be the minimum safe volume that can be left after extended resection in patients with normal liver.

Unfortunately 55–80% of patients resected for colorectal metastases will have a recurrence in one or more sites. One isolated liver relapse develops in 15–40% of these patients, while 25% present with lung and/or abdominal metastases. Only 1/3 of patients with isolated liver relapse are candidates for a potentially curative re-resection. Many investigators have evaluated the possibility and the utility of a second resection to treat hepatic relapses. These studies have demonstrated that long-term survival results after repeated resections (especially in patients with a long disease-free interval between the first and the second resection) are similar to those reported for primary hepatectomies, with a 5-year survival rate which ranges from 30 to 45% [24–29] (Table 6.2). Repeated hepatectomies can provide long-term survival and should be offered to patients based on the same criteria used for initial hepatectomy.

In conclusion surgery remains the only curative treatment for patients with liver metastases from colorectal cancer, being able to offer a 5-year survival higher than 40%. Patients affected by colorectal carcinoma should undergo close follow-up with ultrasonography and tumor marker control, in order to detect a potential liver metastasis at an early stage, allowing the increasing of the resectability. A number of preoperative prognostic factors were detected to help the surgeon in patient selection, but the most important indication is the possibility to obtain a curative resection (R0), sparing a sufficient liver volume.

Furthermore, multimodal therapeutic approache can increase the number of patients who may benefit from surgical treatment and in patients previously considered unresectable gives survival rates similar to those reported for primary resected patients.

Table 6.2 Results after repeated liver resections for colorectal metastases

Author	No.	Perioperative mortality (%)	Survival Median	5-year (%)
Ahmad et al. [24]	19	–	48	44
Morise et al. [25]	30	–	–	30
Fukunaga et al. [26]	11	0.0	28	44
Chiappa et al. [27]	10	0.0	–	44*
Yamada et al. [28]	11	0.0	–	45
Petrowsky et al. [29]	126	1.6	37	34

* 4-year survival

References

1. Simmonds PC, Primrose JN, Colquitt JL et al (2006) Surgical resection of hepatic metastases from colorectal cancer: a systematic review of the published studies. Br J Cancer 94:982–999
2. Jemal A, Siegel R, Ward E et al (2008) Cancer Statistics, 2008. CA Cancer J Clin 58:71–96
3   Pawlik TM, Schulick RD, Choti MA (2008) Expanding criteria for resectability of colorectal liver metastases. Oncologist 13:51–64
4. Schindl M, Wigmore SJ, Currie EJ et al (2005) Prognostic scoring in colorectal cancer liver metastases: development and validation. Arch Surg 140:183–189
5. Wei AC, Greig PD, Grant D et al (2006) Survival after hepatic resection for colorectal metas-

tases: a 10-year experience. Ann Surg Oncol 13:668–676

6. Malik HZ, Prasad KR, Halazun KJ et al (2007) Preoperative prognostic score for predicting survival after hepatic resection for colorectal liver metastases. Ann Surg 246:806–814

7. Arru M, Aldrighetti L, Castoldi R et al (2008) Analysis of prognostic factors influencing long-term survival after hepatic resection for metastatic colorectal cancer. World J Surg 32:93–103

8. Ambiru S, Miyazaki M, Isono T et al (1999) Hepatic resection for colorectal metastases: analysis of prognostic factors. Dis Colon Rectum 42:632–639

9. Nuzzo G, Giulante F, Ardito F et al (2008) Influence of surgical margin on type of recurrence after liver resection for colorectal metastases: a single-center experience. Surgery 143:384–393

10. Laurent C, Sa Cunha A, Couderc P et al (2003) Influence of postoperative morbidity on long-term survival following liver resection for colorectal metastases. Br J Surg 90:1131–1136

11. Viganò L, Ferrero A, Lo Tesoriere R, Capussotti L (2008) Liver surgery for colorectal metastases: results after 10 years of follow-up. long-term survivors, late recurrences, and prognostic role of morbidity. Ann Surg Oncol May 8 [Epub ahead of print].

12. Fong Y, Fortner J, Sun RL et al (1999) Clinical score for predicting recurrence after hepatic resection for metastatic colorectal cancer: analysis of 1001 consecutive cases. Ann Surg 230:309–318

13. Choti MA, Sitzmann JV, Tiburi MF et al (2002) Trends in long-term survival following liver resection for hepatic clorectal metastases. Ann Surg 235:759–766

14. Fernandez FG, Drebin JA, Linehan DC et al (2004) Five-year survival after resection of hepatic metastases from colorectal cancer in patients screened by positron emission tomography with F-18 fluorodeoxyglucose (FDG-PET). Ann Surg 240:438–447

15. Pawlik TM, Scoggins CR, Zorzi D et al (2005) Effect of surgical margin status on survival ad site of recurrence after hepatic resection for colorectal metastases. Ann Surg 241:715–722

16. Guzzetti E, Pulitanò C, Catena M et al (2008) Impact of type of liver resection on the outcome of colorectal liver metastases: a case-matched analysis. J Surg Oncol 97:503–507

17. Helling TS, Blondeau B (2005) Anatomic segmental resection compared to major hepatectomy in the treatment of liver neoplasms. HPB (Oxford) 7:222–225

18. Pawlik TM, Choti MA (2007) Surgical therapy for colorectal metastases to the liver. J Gastrointest Surg 11:1057–1077

19. Covey AM, Brown KT, Jarnagin WR et al (2008) Combined portal vein embolization and neoadjuvant chemotherapy as a treatment strategy for resectable hepatic colorectal metastases. Ann Surg 247:451–455

20. Adam R, Delvart V, Pascal G et al (2004) Rescue surgery for unresectable colorectal liver metastases downstaged by chemotherapy: a model to predict long-term survival. Ann Surg 240:664–657

21. Pawlik TM, Izzo F, Cohen DS et al (2003) Combined resection and radiofrequency ablation for advanced hepatic malignancies: results in 172 patients. Ann Surg Oncol 10:1059–1069

22. Miller G, Biernacki P, Kemeny NE et al (2007) Outcomes after resection of synchronous or metachronous hepatic and pulmonary colorectal metastases. J Am Coll Surg 205:231–238

23. Elias D, Ouellet JF, Bellon N et al (2003) Extrahepatic disease does not contraindicate hepatectomy for colorectal liver metastases. Br J Surg 90:567–574

24. Ahmad A, Chen SL, Bilchik AJ (2007) Role of repeated hepatectomy in the multimodal treatment of hepatic colorectal metastases. Arch Surg 142:526–531

25. Morise Z, Sugioka A, Fujita J et al (2006) Does repeated surgery improve the prognosis of colorectal liver metastases? J Gastrointest Surg 10:6–11

26. Fukunaga K, Takada Y, Otsuka M et al (2003) Resection of localized recurrences after hepatectomy of colorectal cancer metastases. Hepatogastroenterology 50:1894–1897

27. Chiappa A, Zbar AP, Biella F, Staudacher C (1999) Survival after repeat hepatic resection for recurrent colorectal metastase. Hepatogastroenterology 46:1065–1070

28. Yamada H, Katoh H, Kondo S et al (2001) Repeat hepatectomy for recurrent hepatic metastases from colorectal cancer. Hepatogastroenterology 48:828–830
29. Petrowsky H, Gonen M, Jarnagin W et al (2002) Second liver resections are safe and effective treatment for recurrent hepatic metastases from colorectal cancer: a bi-institutional analysis. Ann Surg 235:863–871

Chapter 7

Gastric Cancer

Clemente Iascone, Annalisa Paliotta, Silvia Femia

Gastric cancer is the second most common cancer world-wide, with a frequency that varies greatly across different geographic locations [1]. Its incidence is higher in southern and Eastern Europe; in Italy there are 22.1 new cases/100,000 males and 11.2 cases/100,000 females annually. Gastric cancer is rare before the age of 40, and its incidence peaks in the seventh decade of life. In recent decades the survival rate for gastric cancer has improved in countries such as Japan [2], but in Western countries in patients resected with curative intent the recurrence rate is 40 to 65% [3] and the overall 5-year survival rate is 30% [4, 5]. Differences in the incidence and overall survival of gastric cancer suggest ethnic origin as a possible risk factor [2], but environmental, dietary and behavioral factors may be more relevant than ethnicity with the generation of carcinogenic N-nitroso compounds, while the influence of smoking and alcohol consumption has not been completely clarified [6]. An important development in the epidemiology of gastric carcinoma has been the recognition of the association with *Helicobacter pylori* infection: early infection induces changes in the gastric mucosa with progression to gastric atrophy and intestinal metaplasia predisposing the patient to the development of carcinoma and reducing the risk of duodenal ulcer due to the decreased acid production associated with gastritis. In patients with late *Helicobacter pylori* infection, atrophic gastritis is less frequently observed and therefore the risk of gastric cancer is lower [7], while, in patients with long-lasting reflux disease, antisecretory drugs and eradication of *Helicobacter pylori* infection [8] could increase the incidence of cancer of the gastric cardia [9].

Methods

Patient Population

From 1991 to 2005, 501 patients with gastric adenocarcinoma were admitted to the Department of Surgery "Pietro Valdoni": 420 out of 501 patients underwent resective surgery. Twenty percent of patients were lost at follow-up; in the

A. Bolognese, L. Izzo (eds.), *Surgery in Multimodal Management of Solid Tumors.*
©Springer-Verlag Italia 2009

remaining patients the minimum follow-up was three years and in 80% of subjects it was ten years or longer. Patients were divided according to age into four groups: less than 45 years, 45 to 60 years, 61 to 75 years and above 75 years of age. Clinicopathologic data and patient survival were compared according to age groups and sex. Furthermore, the long-term survival was evaluated in the overall population according to the surgical and adjuvant treatment.

Statistical Evaluation

Data are presented as mean ± standard deviation. Statistical analysis of clinicopathologic factors were analyzed using the "Chi-square test" and "Student T test" assuming as statistically significant $p < 0.05$.

Results

Age and Gender

Four hundred and twenty patients with gastric cancer entered the study; the mean age was 62.4 ±12 years; 6.2% were younger than 45 years; 28.6% were aged 45 to 60 years, 46.4% were aged 61 to 75 years and 18.8% were older than 75 years. Females were more represented in the group of patients over 75 years (26.4% females vs. 14.3% males); males were more frequently observed in the age group 61 to 75 years (51.3% vs. 38%).

Symptoms

At the time of admission, 2.6% of patients were asymptomatic, while in the majority of subjects clinical manifestations occurred as one or two isolated symptoms with an incidence of 92.3% in patients younger than 45 years, 81.7% in patients 45 to 60 years, 74.3% in subjects 61 to 75 years and 83.5% in patients older than 75 years. Epigastric pain was the most common symptom reported by patients, regardless of age: the lowest incidence (50.8%) was reported by patients 61 to75 years, while the highest (69.2%) by patients younger than 45 years.

Surgical Therapy

A "radical" procedure was achieved in 98% of cases; 41.2% of patients underwent total gastrectomy and 58.8% subtotal gastrectomy; both procedures were similarly represented in the four age groups. Reconstruction of digestive continuity was achieved with the Roux-en-Y procedure in patients with total gastrectomy, and with the Billroth II procedure in patients with subtotal or distal gastrectomy. A proximal gastrectomy was required in only a few patients and intestinal continuity was restored by means of an esophagogastrostomy. Overall long-term results were similar for both surgical procedures: 34% of patients after total gastrectomy and 45% after subtotal gastrectomy survived 5 years or longer, 20% of patients after total gastrectomy and 31% after subtotal gastrectomy were alive at 10 years, while almost 14% of patients survived more than 10 years regardless of the surgical therapy.

Tumor Location

More than 80% of tumors were located distally (gastric body, antrum, pyloric/prepyloric area). The incidence of gastric carcinoma of the proximal third, (cardia and/or fundus), increased with increasing patient age: 3.8% in patients younger than 45 years, 15.8% in the 45–60 age group and more than 25% in patients older than 60 years. Overall 5-year survival was 44.5% in patients with lesions of the gastric body and 41.5% in those with antral or pyloric/prepyloric tumors. Patients presenting lesions of the proximal third of the stomach had the worst long-term prognosis, as less than 30% of them were alive at five years from the surgical procedure.

Postoperative Morbidity and Mortality

Increasing age was associated with increased complications and hospital mortality. There were no complications or deaths in the group of patients younger than 45 years. Mortality and morbidity rates were 1.6 and 6.7% in the group of patients aged 45–60, respectively, 3 and 9.2% in the 61–75 age group, and 3.8 and 11.4% in patients older than 75 years.

Primary Tumor and Stage of Disease

Patients younger than 45 years showed the highest rate of both early and late stages, since stage I was diagnosed in 46.1% of them as well as stage III/ IV; intermediate stages, such as Stage II, were more frequently observed in patients older than 60 years. Furthermore, the 38.5% incidence of T1s–T1 in patients younger than 45 years decreased to 15.8, 17.4 and 12.5%, respectively, in patients 45 to 60 years, 61 to 75 years and in those older than 75 years. Advanced T-stage tumors, i.e. T2–T3–T4, were mostly represented in the group of patients over 75 years, with an incidence of 85%. This figure progressively decreased in the remaining three groups. Patients with an early stage of disease showed better long-term prognosis: five-year survival rate was 77% for Stage I patients, 32% for Stage II, 12% for Stage III and 4% for Stage IV. Similarly, five-year survival rate was 84% for Tis or T1 tumors, 35% for T2 lesions and 10 to 15% for T3–T4 cancers.

Survival Analysis and Lymphatic Invasion

Out of 338 patients with gastric cancer, 128 or 37.9% were staged as N0 and 210 or 62.1% showed lymph node involvement (N1–N2–N3). The five-year survival rate was 72.7% in node-negative patients (N0), 30% in patients with N1 involvement, 12.5% in patients with N2 involvement and 0% in patients staged as N3. Furthermore, the 5-year survival rate was 43% when nodal involvement was observed in ≤25% of all nodes examined, 25% when metastasis were present in 25–50% of nodes and only 6% when more than 50% of nodes were involved.

Survival Rate and Histological Classification

Intestinal-type tumors were detected in 51.8% of patients, diffuse-type in 33.4% and a mixed-type in 10.6% of subjects. According to Ming's classification, infiltrative-type tumors were present in 53.2% of patients and expansive-type tumors in 38.5%. In 4.2% of Lauren's classification and in 8.3% of Ming's classification, carcinomas were "not otherwise specified". Lauren "intestinal" type and Ming "expansive" type were associated with the best long-term prognosis as five-year survival rates were 48.6 and 55.4%, respectively. In contrast, when Lauren "diffuse" and "mixed" types or Ming "infiltrative" type were diagnosed, survival was less than 5 years in 70, 69.4 and 73.3% of patients, respectively.

Histological Grading

In patients younger than 45 years, the incidence of G1 and G2 tumors was 27% while it was 32.5, 42.6 and 46.8%, respectively, in patients aged 45 to 60 years, 61 to 75 years and in those older than 75 years. In contrast, the incidence of undifferentiated cancers was 69.2% in patients younger than 45 years and 65.8% in those aged 45 to 60 years. The overall 5-year survival rate was 89% in patients with differentiated tumors (G1), 42.2% in patients with moderately differentiated type (G2) and 31.7% in patients with the undifferentiated type (G3).

Survival and Adjuvant Therapy

Three-year survival rates were 57.9% in female patients and 50.4% in male patients regardless of the type of surgery performed and staging of disease. Most deaths for both males and females were registered in the first two years of follow-up as the mortality rate was 15–20% and lowered to 5–6% a year over the subsequent follow-up period. Survival rates were higher in females than in males with differences ranging from 5 to 7% per year in favor of female patients; however at ten years from surgery, overall survival rates were similar for both females and males and were 21 and 19%, respectively (Fig. 7.1). Following surgery, adjuvant chemotherapy was performed in 71 (21%) patients, while 267 patients were treated with surgery alone: when the survival curves of these groups were compared, patients as combined treatment showed a better outcome than patients with surgery alone, with survival rates from the first to the fourth year of follow-up were 95.8, 77.5, 66.2, 52.2%. The corresponding figures for patients with surgery alone were 77.1, 60.3, 49.4 and 43% indicating a survival advantage of surgery plus adjuvant chemotherapy ranging from 11 to 17%. From the fifth year of follow-up survival curves were similar for both groups of patients, as differences, even though present, were less remarkable and ranged from 2 to 5% (Fig. 7.2).

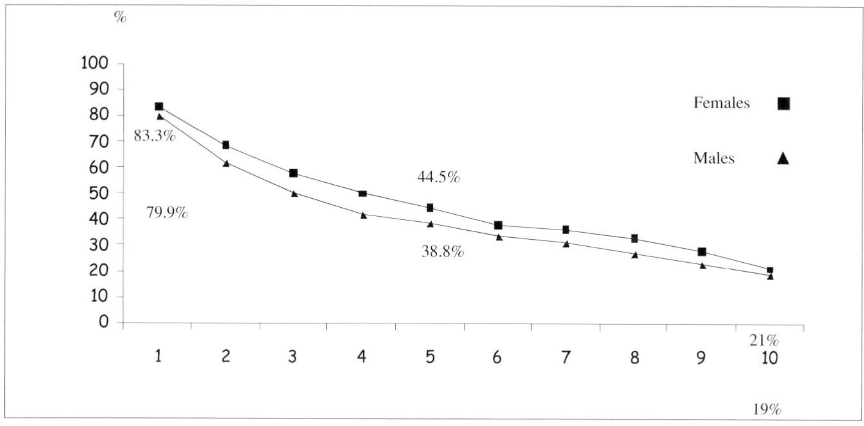

Fig. 7.1 Gastric cancer (1991-2005) survival curves

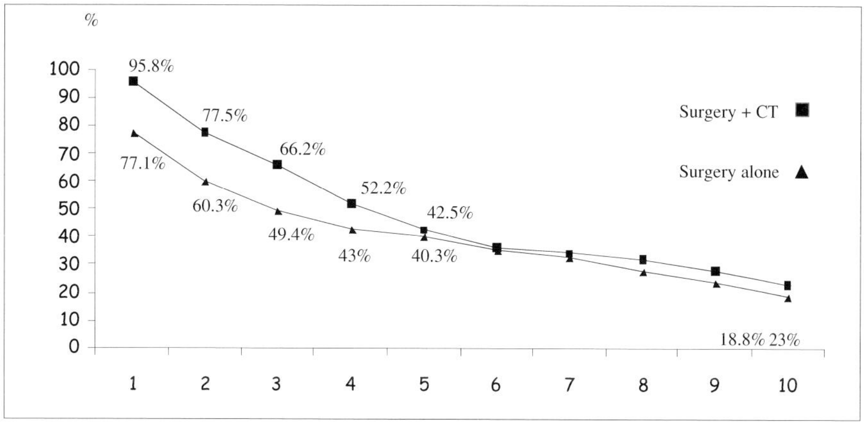

Fig. 7.2 Gastric cancer (1991–2005) survival curves: surgery +CT vs. surgery alone

Discussion

Despite the decreasing worldwide incidence in the last 50 years, gastric cancer accounts for 3 to 10% of all cancer-related deaths. The results of our study support similar epidemiologic observations in Western countries [10] and has documented that 70% of patients with gastric cancer, even though with some differences between males and females, are older than 65 years reflecting the aging of the population. As women live longer, they are more likely to develop the disease than men. Moreover, total mortality and morbidity increase gradually with the age of patients regardless of sex. In elderly patients, the incidence of post-surgical mortality and morbidity are double or triple than that of young patients. This increased number of complications may be attributable to several associated diseases in elderly patients, such as blood hypertension, cardiac or cerebrovascular diseases, anemia, respiratory problems and hypoalbuminemia. These comorbid conditions have been found in over 50% of older patients, thus indicating that age may be a confounding factor and its influence is not of independent prognostic value; age when associated with known risk factors that can significantly affect the patient's clinical course can be identified as a significant prognostic variable. These observations support some surgical trends aimed "to tailor" the operative procedure according to patient age and clinical condition. More aggressive and extended treatments should be performed in younger patients whereas more conservative procedures may be more suitable for the oldest, as the main concern for the elderly should be more centered on quality of life rather than cancer eradication. To this end, the results of our study do not show long-term survival advantages to support extended resections and confirm previous observations [11]. A recently published prospective study failed to show any statistically significant difference in 10-year survival rates after total or subtotal gastrectomy. Furthermore, in our series the 5-year survival rate of 34.1% after total gastrectomy is lower than the 44.3% after subtotal gastrectomy. These findings are consistent with the 5-year survival rate of 32.4% after total gastrectomy reported in a recently published study of 1,114 patients with gastric cancer [10]. In addition, in patients with cancer of the gastric antrum, similar 5- and 10-year survival rates have been documented after subtotal or total gastrectomy. On the other hand, the location of the primary tumor is itself a prognostic factor that can influence long-term survival: cancers of the gastric body or gastric antrum showed the same 40–45% 5-year survival rate, which was higher than the 29% survival rate achieved for carcinomas of the upper third of the stomach. This observation supports some data of the literature that identify proximal location as a negative prognostic factor on long-term survival when compared with more distal gastric cancers [10]. In this study on more than 18,000 patients with gastric cancer, the long-term survival was 15–18% for cancer of the proximal third of the stomach regardless of the type of resection performed, 38% after subtotal gastrectomy and 31% after total gastrectomy for tumors of the gastric body, while antral cancers seemed to benefit from total gastrectomy compared to subtotal gastrectomy as long-term survival rates were respectively 34 and 26%.

Intestinal type adenocarcinomas are more frequently observed and arise in areas where the normal gastric mucosa is replaced by intestinal metaplasia: intestinal type tumors are associated with 49% 5-year survival rate, while in diffuse and mixed type adenocarcinoma the survival rate is 29–30%. The diffuse type of cancer is usually more represented in Western series, while the intestinal type is more common in Japan. Our own results and data from the literature indicate that diffuse-type lesions are associated with a worse long term prognosis than intestinal type tumors: Wanebo et al. [10] reported 23% survival rate for the intestinal type tumors, 10% for the diffuse type and 18% for the mixed type. This finding and the prevalence of intestinal type tumors in Japanese patients may explain the different results between Western and Japanese series. Furthermore, the results of our study show that the degree of cell differentiation ("grading") was able to influence the long-term survival of the patient. Thus well differentiated tumors (G1) were associated with a better long-term survival, supporting the findings of various studies which show that long-term survival is statistically different between patients with well or poorly differentiated tumors. The long term survival of patients operated on for gastric cancer is largely related to TNM stage of cancer at the time of resection and to the primary tumor (T) and nodal involvement (N) as independent risk factors [10, 11]. In our series, stage I and T1 patients showed 73 and 84% 5-year survival rates, respectively. For stage II and T2 lesions survival rates decreased to 32 and 36%, and for stage III/IV and T3/T4 lesions the rates were 4–16%. The results of our study are comparable to those reported by studies performed in Western countries [11]. By comparing the data obtained from a large North American study with those of 56 Japanese centers [10], it has been shown that the incidence of stage I tumors is significantly higher in Japanese series than in the American series, where stage III/IV are largely more represented: the overall more favorable long-term results reported by Japanese authors compared to other investigations carried out in Western countries may be accounted for by the marked prevalence of less advanced diseases usually observed in the Asian series [10]. However, it must be underlined that better results were also reported by Asian authors even though Japanese and Western patients were compared by stage: more accurate resections of the primary tumor and more extended lymphadenectomies may play a role in achieving these results. Japanese investigators assert that the extended lymphadenectomy removes tumor in the regional lymph nodes before they can metastasize. In addition it is argued that extended lymphadenectomy improves staging accuracy. The role of nodal involvement as an important prognostic variable has been documented in our study as well: patient survivals greater than 5 years were observed in 73% of patients classified as N0 and in 30% of patients classified as N1. Similarly, "the overall amount" of nodes involved has an impact on long-term survival, since in patients with no more than 25% of nodes involved the survival rate was 42%, while it was 4–12% when 50% or more of nodes were involved. Our findings are consistent with those of several studies reporting a 10-year survival rate of 70% for patients classified as N0, 41% for N1 and less than 20% for N2–N3 [11]. Over the past twenty years the overall survival in patients undergoing surgical treatment for gastric cancer has gradually improved not only in Asia but also in Europe and North America. A recent review [11] covering a twenty-year period documented an improvement in 5-year survival from 15 to 41% with an increase in curative resections from 33 to 73%. Similar results have been reported in studies from Germany and the United States [11]. Our data confirm this trend, with a global survival at 3 years of 58% in females and 50.4% in males and, respectively, 44.5 and 38.8% at 5 years, comparable with the results reported above. A further improvement of long-term prognosis could be achieved by appropriate adjuvant and/or neoadjuvant therapy, although to date no studies have ever documented any benefit of such therapies in patients operated upon for gastric cancer [11]. In our study, 71 patients were submitted to adjuvant chemotherapy. The results observed comparing patients treated with surgery and chemotherapy to patients undergoing surgical treatment alone indicate in the first 4 years of follow-up an improvement in terms of survival rates in subjects submitted to adjuvant chemotherapy with a "gain" in percentage terms of 17–18% in the first three years and 11% in the fourth year, while from the fifth to the tenth year of follow-up, the survival curves of both groups of patients are similar. The better outcome documented in the first half of the follow-up period in patients submitted to adjuvant chemotherapy cannot be clearly explained. Since 15-20% of patients die early in the follow-up, some of them may benefit from adjuvant chemotherapy, therefore "recruiting" to survival patients who otherwise would die in the 24 months following surgery alone. However, patients enrolled in the present study were managed by several surgeons and the choice of adjuvant treatment and type of chemotherapy regimen were the result of the individual surgeon's clinical behavior and personal viewpoint. Therefore, the results we observed, even though encouraging, must be interpreted with caution and require further investigations and rigorous evaluation.

References

1. Bozzetti F, Marubini E, Bonfanti G et al (1999) Subtotal versus total gastrectomy for gastric cancer: five year survival rates in a multicenter randomized Italian trial. Italian Gastrointestinal Tumor Study Group. Ann Surg 230:170–178
2. Davis P, Takeshi S (2001) The difference in gastric cancer between Japan, USA, and Europe: what are the facts? What are the suggestions? Crit Rev Oncol Hematol 40:77–94
3. MacDonald J, Smalley S, Benedetti J et al (2001) Chemioradiotherapy after surgery compared with surgery alone for adenocarcinoma of the stomach or gastroesophageal junction. N Engl J Med 345:725–729
4. Doglietto G, Pacelli F, Caprino P et al (2000) Surgery: independent prognostic factor in curable and far advanced gastric cancer. World J Surg 24:459–464
5. Hartgrink H, Putter H, Kranenbarg E et al (2002) Value of palliative resection in gastric cancer, Br J Surg 89:1438–1443
6. Devisa S, Blot W, Fraumeni J (1998) Changing patterns in the incidence of esophageal and gastric carcinoma in the US. Cancer 83:2049–2053
7. Uemura N, Okamoto S, Yamamoto S et al (2001) Helicobacter pylori infection and the development of gastric cancer. N Engl J Med 345:784–789

8. Lagergreen J, Bergstrom R (1999) Association between body mass and adenocarcinoma of the oesophagus and gastric cardia. Ann Intern Med 130:883–890
9. Lagergreen J, Bergstrom R (1999) Symptomatic gastro-esophageal reflux as a risk factor for esophageal adenocarcinoma. N Engl J Med 340:825–831
10. Wanebo HJ, Kennedy BJ, Chmiel J et al (1993) Cancer of the stomach. A patient care study by the American college   of Surgeons. Ann Surg 218(5):583–592
11. Brennan MF (2005) Current status of surgery for gastric cancer: a review. Gastric Cancer 8:64–70

Chapter 8

Cancer of the Exocrine Pancreas: Surgery and Multimodal Treatment

Giuliano Barugola, Massimo Falconi, Fabio Zarantonello, Giuseppe Malleo, Claudio Bassi, Paolo Pederzoli

Introduction

The optimal management of pancreatic ductal carcinoma remains poorly defined. Radical resection is possible in about 20–30% of patients, with an overall 5-year survival rate of only 20% [1]. In recent years, perioperative morbidity and mortality have significantly decreased, and different clinical trials have suggested an important role for adjuvant therapy [2].

Prior to the 1990s, the results of resective surgery were disappointing: recurrence of disease was almost the rule and even short-term survival rates were dismal, mainly due to surgery-related morbidity and mortality [3]. The first attempts at improving surgical outcome included extended resections, up to total pancreatectomy, and extended lymphadenectomy [4, 5]. However, the results did not meet the expectations, as these procedures were associated with an increase in short- and long-term postoperative complications and a deterioration in quality of life [6].

The introduction of intravenous systemic gemcitabine has radically changed ductal carcinoma management, particularly with regard to clinician mentality. Gemcitabine treatment has shown a significant, but unfortunately not dramatic, increase in survival in advanced disease, with a substantial improvement in quality of life [7]. Accordingly, it has become the standard treatment of unresectable patients. While on the one hand these results are of great importance from a strictly oncologic point of view, on the other they have also led to a change in mentality towards a multidisciplinary approach for resected patients.

Actually, adjuvant therapy combined with chemoradiation has already been a part of clinical practice in highly specialized centers, despite the lack of evidence with regard to its safety and efficacy. The GITSG (Gastrointestinal Tumor Study Group) study showed that radiotherapy combined with 5-fluorouracil (5-FU) chemotherapy prolonged survival rates following apparent curative resection [8]. However, these results were not confirmed in a second large European study. The EORTC (European Organisation for Research and Treatment of Cancer) trial, published in 1999, concluded that the addition of chemoradiation plus chemotherapy (5-FU given during radiation for 5 days) to surgery did not

A. Bolognese, L. Izzo (eds.), *Surgery in Multimodal Management of Solid Tumors.*
©Springer-Verlag Italia 2009

produce any benefit in resected pancreatic cancer patients [9]. Other types of antitumoral approaches with a minor systemic impact have also been proposed, but neither intraoperative radiotherapy (IORT) nor locoregional chemotherapy have shown any clear advantages in terms of overall survival or disease-free interval [10, 11]. These attempts, however, opened the way to large scale randomized studies both in the adjuvant and, more recently, neoadjuvant setting [12]. Much effort has been spent in our national referral center for improving the prognosis of resected and/or resectable pancreatic carcinoma. In this light, the aim of the present chapter is to report changes and results obtained in our center, taking into account the still-existing open questions on the multimodal approach to the disease.

Institutional Experience

Population and Perioperative Work-up

From 1990 to 2006, 409 patients with histologically proven pancreatic ductal carcinoma were resected at the Department of Surgery of the University of Verona. The diagnostic work-up included at least a computed tomography and/or magnetic resonance scan, a transabdominal ultrasound (with contrast medium since 2002) and laboratory tests including CEA (n.v. <5 ng/mL) and Ca 19-9 (n.v. <25 U/mL). Resection was undertaken according to the site of the disease, when pre- and intraoperative exploration confirmed any of the following findings: (1) the lack of infiltration of arterial vessels, but splenic artery 1 cm far from celiac trunk; (2) the lack of complete infiltration of venous vessels or an encasement of more than 180 circumferential degrees and/or more than 1.5 cm in length; (3) the lack of any distant spread. Table 8.1 reports the main characteristics, clinical and laboratory data of the study population. The diagnosis was mostly sign/symptoms-related. Jaundice and pain made up the main complaints in 58.6 and 43% of cases, respectively. Only 32 individuals (7.8%) were incidentally diagnosed. All the patients were monitored on a 3-month basis after resection through imaging and laboratory tests. Follow-up was updated at least until December 2007.

Type of Operation and Surgical Results

The type of surgical procedures, main intra- and peri-operative data are summarized in Table 8.2. Overall, 321 (78.4%) pancreaticoduodenectomies were carried out. The pancreatic remnant was always anastomosed to either a jejunal loop (286 cases; 89%) or the stomach (35 cases; 11%). Total pancreatectomy was performed in 15 patients (4.6%) with positive resection margins (frozen section) and when the general conditions were good enough to manage the subsequent endocrine and exocrine insufficiency. Standard lymphadenectomy was the

Table 8.1 Main characteristics, clinical and laboratory data of 409 patients resected for pancreatic cancer from 1990 to 2006 at the Department of Surgery of Verona University

	Patients	%
Sex (male/female)	239/170	
Age (years)*	63	IQR (35–79)
Symptoms at diagnosis		
– Jaundice	240	58.6
– Weight loss >3 kg	223	54.4
– Pain	176	43.0
Duration of symptoms (days)	30	IQR (14–94)
Incidental diagnosis	32	7.8
CEA (ng/mL)*	2.4	IQR (1–5)
Ca19-9 (U/mL)*	105	IQR (11–320)

* Median
IQR, Interquartile range

Table 8.2 Type of operation and perioperative data in 409 patients resected for pancreatic cancer from 1990 to 2006 at the Department of Surgery of Verona University

	Patients	%
Type of operation		
– Pylorus preserving PD	245	60.0
– Whipple PD	76	18.4
– Left pancreatectomy	73	17.0
– Total pancreatectomy	15	4.6
– Vascular resection	32	7.8
Operative data		
– Operative time (min)*	360	IQR (240-500)
– Blood transfusion (patients)*	0	IQR (0-2)
– Hospital stay (days)*	12	IQR (6-20)
Main postoperative complications		
– Abdominal	131	32
– Pancreatic fistula	74	18
Reoperations	20	4.8
Mortality	4	0.9

* Median
PD, Pancreaticoduodenectomy; *IQR*, interquartile range

rule, except in 32 patients (7.8%) who were randomized to extended lymphadenectomy, according to a specific trial [13]. Thirty-two patients (7.8%) underwent vascular resection in an attempt to achieve an R-0 resection. With regard to postoperative course, 131 patients (32%) faced an abdominal complication, mainly related to the development of pancreatic fistula (18% of cases). Twenty patients (4.8%) underwent a re-operation, mainly due to bleeding. Median hospital stay was 12 days, which significantly decreased over time. It was in fact 16 days from 1990 to 1999, 12 days from 2000 to 2003 and 8 days in the last period, respectively (p <0.001). Over the years, the proportion of patients older than 70 years undergoing resection has significantly increased. Considering the same periods, their percentage was 17, 26 and 31%, respectively (p <0.001). Thirty-day postoperative mortality was 0.9% (4 patients). Three of them were reoperated. In two cases repeat laparotomy was undertaken for bleeding due to severe postoperative pancreatitis, and in one case due to an infected collection. One patient died of a heart attack on postoperative day 2.

Pathologic Results

Intraoperative frozen exam of the surgical resection margins was routinely performed. Whenever positive, the resection was enlarged. Once the resection is completed, the pathologic protocol foresees a first macroscopic examination with recognition of all the surgical "classical" margins, as well as the retroperitoneal margin. The latter (the fibrotic tissue between the pancreas and the superior mesenteric artery) has been colored in Indian ink since 1997. The specimens are then fixed in formalin and afterwards entirely microscopically examined through mapping samples. T, N and grading are assessed. Grading was scored as G1 (well differentiated), G2 (moderate), G3 (poorly differentiated) and anaplastic (G4). All cases were restaged according to the 2002 UICC classification [14]. Quality of resection was determined according to the R-classification by the International Union Against Cancer (R0 = no residual tumor, R1 = all identifiable tumor removed but tumor cells are present at ≤1 mm from any aforementioned surgical margin, R2 = tumor left macroscopically *in situ*). One hundred-six patients (26%) had an R1 resection, mainly related to a microscopic positive retroperitoneal margin (67 cases; 64%). Table 8.3 summarizes the main post resectional pathologic parameters.

Multidisciplinary Approach

Two-hundred fifty-two (61.6%) patients received an adjuvant treatment, which consisted in chemotherapy in 168 patients (66.7%) and in chemoradiation therapy in the remaining 84. In the earlier period (until 1994) all the resected patients did not have any adjuvant treatment following resection (n = 34). In the second period (1995 to 2006), most of the patients were enrolled and random-

Table 8.3 Main pathological features of 409 patients resected for pancreatic cancer from 1990 to 2006 at the Department of Surgery of Verona university

	Patients	%
Resection margin		
R0	259	63.3
R1	106	26.0
R2	44	10.7
Tumor size (mm)*	29	IQR (18-41)
Node positive	309	75.5
Grading		
G1	20	4.8
G2	239	58.4
G3	140	34.3
G4	10	2.5
Stage UICC 2002		
Ia	12	2.9
Ib	2	0.6
IIa	85	20.7
IIb	271	66.3
III	26	6.3
IV	13	3.2

*Median
IQR, Interquartile range

ized into different ongoing trials (ESPAC-1 [15] and then ESPAC-3 [16]. In particular, 50 patients (12.2%) were enrolled in the ESPAC-1 trial and randomly assigned to chemotherapy (5- FU at the dose of 425 mg/m^2 in bolus, 5 days every 28 days x 6 cycles, plus folinic acid [FA] at a dose of 20 mg/m^2) versus chemoradiotherapy alone (20 Gy twice over a two-week period plus 5-FU). The remaining patients were assigned to a chemoradiotherapy regimen associated with chemotherapy or to observation. A further 41 patients (10.8%) were enrolled in the ESPAC-3 trial and randomized to receive either the same chemotherapeutic regimen as the ESPAC-1 trial or gemcitabine (1,000 mg/m^2 weekly for 3 weeks out of every 4 weeks for 6 months).

Since 1995, the main reasons for not being submitted to adjuvant therapy were: (a) randomization in the observation arm of the ESPAC-1 trial ($n = 25$) or (b) an insufficient or late (8 weeks) recovery after surgery. So far, the distribution of patients who received or not a treatment before or, mainly, after surgery was significantly different ($p < 0.005$) over the years, as reported in Fig. 8.1.

Regarding patients older than 70 years, the percentage of those receiving adjuvant treatment increased from 10% (period 1995–1999) to 56% (period 2004-2006) (p <0.001). In the latter period, 15 patients (3.6%) were resected after neo-adjuvant treatment (Fig. 8.1). The decision was outside any specific protocol, according to the referring surgeon and after informed consent.

Overall median survival was 18.5 months (C.I. 95% 16.9–21.3), with a 5-year survival rate of 18.3% (Fig. 8.2). Multimodal treatment (radical surgery combined with adjuvant chemotherapy or chemoradiotherapy) offered the longest life expectancy (median: 20.4 months C.I. 95% 18.7–23.2) compared with surgery alone (median: 17.6 months C.I. 95% 16.7–20.7) (p <0.0005) (Fig. 8.3).

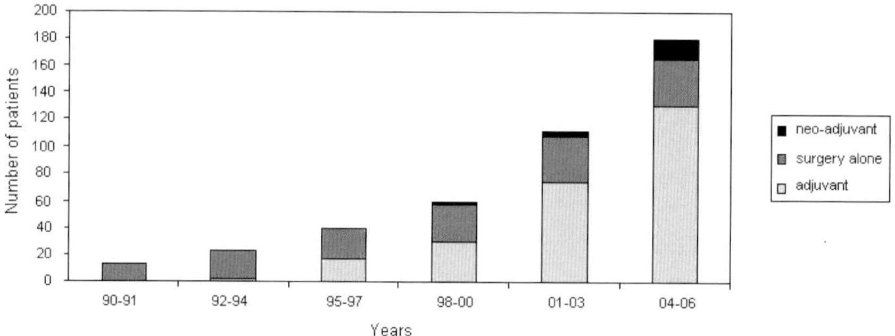

Fig. 8.1 Changes toward a multimodal approach in resected patients for ductal carcinoma over the years 1990–2006 at the Surgical Department of Verona University

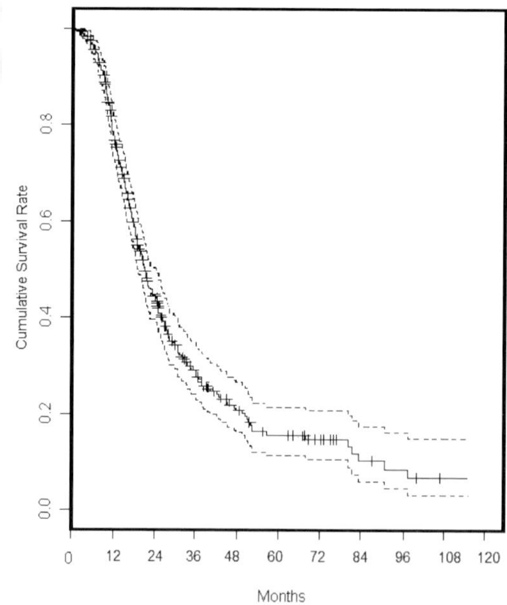

Fig. 8.2 Overall survival of the 409 patients resected for ductal carcinoma from 1990 to 2006 at the Surgical Department of Verona University (median: 18.5 months; C.I. 95% 16.9–21.3)

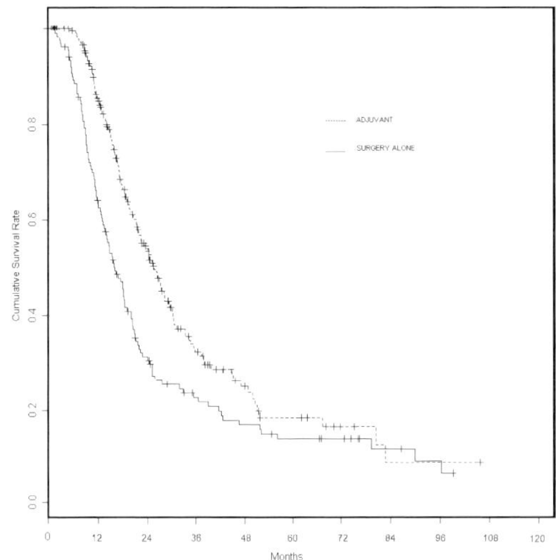

Fig. 8.3 Kaplan-Meier survival curves of resected patients for ductal carcinoma who underwent surgery alone (median: 17.6 months C.I. 95% 16.7–20.7) or adjuvant treatments (chemo- and/or chemoradiotherapy) (median: 20.4 months C.I. 95% 18.7–23.2) ($p < 0.0005$)

Discussion

The affirmation, often quoted prior to 1995, that "surgery is the only chance for the cure of patients with pancreatic cancer" has proven to be inappropriate. In fact, despite an apparently curative surgical approach, the disease usually recurs. Ninety-five percent of tumors relapse within 2 years from their resection, and the most common sites of failure (97%) are intra-abdominal [17]. These include the surgical bed, the liver and the peritoneal cavity. Five-year survival ranges from 5 to 25% of cases. These figures have led in recent years to a more accurate affirmation stating that "resection is only the first step towards long-term survival". This simple statement is the result of a long journey, which has gathered together many different lessons learned over the last 20 years, between attempts, failures and successes.

Lessons Learned about Surgery

The removal of a pancreatic tumor remains the main procedure aimed at achieving a definitive cure. In order to achieve better local control, two main methods have been experimented in the 1990s. Despite the initial expectations, total pancreatectomy failed to show any advantage over partial resection in terms of both survival and recurrence [18]. In contrast, pylorus-preserving pancreaticoduodenectomy (PPPD) when compared to the classical Whipple procedure guaranteed better metabolic function, hormonal regulation and quality of life, without compromising oncologic radicality, survival, type and incidence of recurrence [19, 20]. Today, in our institution, the Whipple procedure is only carried out for tumors involving the first portion of the duodenum.

In order to reduce local recurrence, another surgical approach has been adopted by extending the lymphadenectomy. Of particular note, the former is invariably linked with increased postoperative morbidity, and impairs quality of life [21]. Quality of life has become of paramount importance, since adjuvant treatment has been shown to increase survival (see below). The current literature shows that a relevant factor in determining the outcome after surgical resection is the experience of both the surgeon and the whole team looking after the patient. There is, in fact, an opposite correlation between the morbidity and the mortality observed, especially after pancreaticoduodenectomy, and the number of patients resected per year [17].

Lesson Learned about Pre- and Peri-resectional Results: the "R Factor"

Incomplete resections (R1 and R2) might be due to three possible factors:
- Poor patient selection, as the result of inadequate preoperative imaging and/or interpretation
- The surgeon's failure to divide the specimen from the retroperitoneum along the peri-adventitial plane of the superior mesenteric artery
- Infiltrative nature of ductal pancreatic carcinoma, as a result of its aggressiveness

The current literature no longer justifies an R2 resection preoperatively planned since the operating time, hospital stay, intraoperative blood loss and severe surgical complications were significantly more frequent after palliative demolition [22]. No definitive significant differences regarding survival were found between R2 resected patients and patients with an advanced disease treated conservatively.

There are no significant differences in survival between R0 and R1 resections. However, some data in the literature suggest that the "R factor" might influence the type of postoperative adjuvant treatment. A recent meta-analysis demonstrated that chemotherapy did not appear to be as effective in the R1 subgroup, mimicking the effect of chemoradiotherapy in the R0 subgroup. Additional controlled trials are needed to find better treatments in patients with R1 resections for ductal carcinoma of the pancreas [23].

Lesson Learned about Survival and Multimodal Treatment

In recent years the role of adjuvant chemotherapy has been definitively assessed. Two European randomized trials have already shown that a 6-month adjuvant treatment course with 5-FU plus FA [16] or gemcitabine [24] is able to offer a significant advantage with regard to overall survival and time to recurrence. The possible role of chemoradiotherapy is still under investigation, even though it is the current adjuvant treatment in the United States despite the results of the ESPAC-1 trial. Novel modalities in delivering radiotherapy should probably be applied and investigated in new randomized trials, selecting R1 resected patients for whom local recurrence control might represent a primary target.

Although radical surgery combined with adjuvant chemotherapy offers the longest life expectancy, overall survival remains gloomy, with an actuarial 5-year rate ranging from 15 to 30%. However, these percentages do not completely represent the disease trend after resection. In fact, up to 20% of resected patients eventually die of disease within 1 year from the resection, regardless of any adjuvant treatment. This is one of the strong motivations for looking at new approaches. Up to now, no randomized controlled trials have been performed to compare neoadjuvant therapy (chemotherapy or chemoradiation) with upfront surgery followed by adjuvant treatment. Data from retrospective analyses and several phase I/II trials [25] seem to demonstrate a potential role of neoadjuvant chemoradiation. The use of a neoadjuvant approach to pancreatic cancer is advocated for its potential ability to (1) optimize the selection of patients who eventually benefit from resective surgery, thereby excluding those with an aggressive and rapidly progressive disease; (2) reduce the number of patients with positive microscopic margins near the mesenteric vessels; (3) decrease the number of cases with nodal involvement, which is a well known adverse prognostic factor; (4) allow the administration of an antitumoral treatment to all resected patients. In this regard, it should be borne in mind that up to 25% of patients (as in our experience) cannot receive adjuvant treatment for an incomplete or late recovery after resection, mainly due to postoperative complications. Another potential advantage of neoadjuvant treatment is the possibility of increasing the number of resected patients through the down-staging of locally advanced tumors, even if only in a small proportion of patients [26].

Novel therapeutic strategies, together with a better understanding of tumor biology, are needed in order to develop pre- and postoperative individualized treatments.

New Treatment and Hopes

Immunotherapy

Immunotherapy is a novel approach which affects the regulation of immune responses by targeting pancreatic-cancer-associated antigens and regulatory signaling molecules. It includes peptide vaccinations, nonspecific immunotherapy, allogene modified tumor cell vaccines, and vector-based vaccines. Although several trials have shown detectable immune responses and some have reported prolonged survival for immune responders, immunotherapy remains experimental. However, some approaches have made it into a phase III setting [27]. In addition, the emerging concept of tumor stem cells may lead to a new focus on immunotherapy, since these often highly chemotherapy-resistant cells are thought to be the source of recurrences.

Pancreatic Cancer Stem Cells

The cancer stem cell hypothesis suggests that neoplastic clones are maintained exclusively by a small subset of cells with stem cell properties within a tumor. There has been strong evidence to support this theory in blood, brain, and breast cancers. Pilot studies are currently underway to investigate pancreatic cancer stem cells. The information gained may lead to new avenues for identifying novel tumor cell markers for diagnostic purposes and to identify new cellular targets, and will provide a cell population that can be used for testing new chemotherapeutic agents, biological modifiers, and immune-based therapies [28].

Gene Therapy

Gene therapy involves the transfer of genetic constructs that alter the neoplastic potential of the cancer cells. Once genetic transfer has developed, the expression of the gene product may modify the biological behavior of the tumor. The first clinical trial of gene therapy conducted to assess its safety and efficacy was conducted in 21 patients with locally advanced pancreatic cancer [29]. Viral vectors were delivered directly within the tumor, and patients received intravenous systemic gemcitabine. There were some severe side-effects in this study, including bacterial infections, which were felt to be secondary to the EUS-guided injection, and duodenal perforation in two patients. No convincing evidence to prove the efficacy of this approach was found.

Interferon-alpha

Alternate adjuvant therapies have also been investigated. Picozzi et al performed a phase II trial of an interferon-based chemotherapy regimen with concomitant postoperative adjuvant radiotherapy [30]. The actuarial overall 1-, 2-, and 5-year survival rates were 95, 64, and 55%, respectively. Although the potential survival benefit with this regimen seems promising, about 70% of the patients developed moderate to severe gastrointestinal toxicity. The confirmatory studies are underway.

References

1. Picozzi VJ, Pisters PW, Vickers SM, Strasberg SM (2008) Strength of the evidence: adjuvant therapy for resected pancreatic cancer. J Gastrointest Surg 12(4):657–661

2. Saif MW (2007) Controversies in the adjuvant treatment of pancreatic adenocarcinoma. JOP 8(5):545–52
3. Bramhall SR, Allum WH, Jones AG et al (1995) Treatment and survival in 13,560 patients with pancreatic cancer, and incidence of the disease, in the West Midlands: an epidemiological study. Br J Surg 82(1):111–115
4. Kayahara M, Nagakawa T, Ueno K et al (1993) An evaluation of radical resection for pancreatic cancer based on the mode of recurrence as determinant by autopsy and diagnostic imaging. Cancer 72:2118–2123
5. Bassi C, Salvia R, Butturini G et al (2005) Value of regional lymphadenectomy in pancreatic cancer. HPB 7(2):87–92
6. Kennedy EP, Yeo CJ (2007) Pancreaticoduodenectomy with extended retroperitoneal lymphadenectomy for periampullary adenocarcinoma. Surg Oncol Clin N Am 16(1):157–176
7. Burris HA 3rd, Moore MJ, Andersen J et al (1997) Improvements in survival and clinical benefit with gemcitabine as first-line therapy for patients with advanced pancreas cancer: a randomized trial. J Clin Oncol 15(6):2403–2413
8. Oettle H, Neuhaus P (2007) Adjuvant therapy in pancreatic cancer: a critical appraisal. Drugs 67(16):2293–2310
9. Klinkenbijl JH, Jeekel J, Sahmoud T et al (1999) Adjuvant radiotherapy and 5-fluorouracil after curative resection of cancer of the pancreas and periampullary region: phase III trial of the EORTC gastrointestinal tract cancer cooperative group. Ann Surg 230(6):776–782
10. Ruano-Ravina A, Almazán Ortega R, Guedea F (2008) Intraoperative radiotherapy in pancreatic cancer: a systematic review. Radiother Oncol [Epub ahead of print]
11. Ishikawa T (2007) Is it relevant that intra-arterial chemotherapy may be effective for advanced pancreatic cancer? World J Gastroenterol 13(32):4306–4309
12. Hoffman JP, Lipsitz S, Pisansky T et al (1998) Phase II trial of preoperative radiation therapy and chemotherapy for patients with localized, resectable adenocarcinoma of the pancreas: an Eastern Cooperative Oncology Group Study. J Clin Oncol 16(1):317–323
13. Pedrazzoli S, Pasquali C, Sperti C (2002) Extent of lymphadenectomy in the resection of pancreatic cancer. Analysis of the existing evidence. Rocz Akad Med Bialymst 50:85–90
14. Greene FL, Page DL, Fleming ID et al (eds) (2002) AJCC Cancer Staging Manual, 6th edn. Springer, New York, pp 157–164
15. Anonymous (2004) ESPAC-3(v2). Phase III Adjuvant trial in pancreatic cancer comparing 5-FU and DL Folinic Acid vs. Gemcitabine. National Cancer Research Network, Trials Portfolio, available at: http://public.ukcrn.org.uk/search/StudyDetail.aspx?StudyID=669
16. Neoptolemos JP, Stocken DD, Friess H et al (2004) A randomized trial of chemoradiotherapy and chemotherapy after resection of pancreatic cancer. N Engl J Med 350(12):1200–1210
17. Barugola G, Falconi M, Bettini R et al (2007) The determinant factors of recurrence following resection for ductal pancreatic cancer. JOP 8(1 Suppl):132–140
18. Westerdahl J, Andren-Sandberg A, Ihse I (1993) Recurrence of exocrine pancreatic cancer – local or hepatic? Hepatogastroenterology 40(4):384–387
19. Lim JE, Chien MW, Earle CC (2003) Prognostic factors following curative resection for pancreatic adenocarcinoma: a population-based, linked database analysis of 396 patients. Ann Surg 237(1):74–85
20. Klinkenbijl JH, van der Schelling GP, Hop WC et al (1992) The advantages of pylorus-preserving pancreatoduodenectomy in malignant disease of the pancreas and periampullary region. Ann Surg 216(2):142–145
21. Kleeff J, Michalski C, Friess H, Buchler MW (2006) Pancreatic cancer: from bench to 5-year survival. Pancreas 33(2):111–118
22. Köninger J, Wente MN, Müller-Stich BP et al (2008) R2 resection in pancreatic cancer –does it make sense? Langenbecks Arch Surg [Epub ahead of print]
23. Butturini G, Stocken DD, Moritz N et al (2008) Influence of resection margins and treatment on survival in patients with pancreatic cancer. Meta-analysis of randomized controlled trials. Arch Surg 143(1):75–83

24. Oettle H, Neuhaus P (2007)Adjuvant therapy in pancreatic cancer: a critical appraisal. Drugs 67(16):2293–2310
25. Evans DB, for The Multidisciplinary Pancreatic Cancer Study Group (2006) Resectable pancreatic cancer: the role for neoadjuvant/preoperative therapy. HPB (Oxford) 8(5):365–368
26. Greer SE, Pipas JM, Sutton JE et al (2008) Effect of neoadjuvant therapy on local recurrence after resection of pancreatic adenocarcinoma. J Am Coll Surg 206(3):451–457
27. Stieler J (2008) Immunotherapeutic approaches in pancreatic cancer. Recent results. Cancer Res 177:165–177
28. Demirer T, Barkholt L, Blaise D et al (2008) Solid Tumors Working Party. Transplantation of allogeneic hematopoietic stem cells: an emerging treatment modality for solid tumors. Nat Clin Pract Oncol [Epub ahead of print]
29. Hecht JR, Bedford R, Abbruzzese JL et al (2003) A phase I/II trial of intratumoral endoscopic ultrasound injection of ONYX-015 with intravenous gemcitabine in unresectable pancreatic carcinoma. Clin Cancer Res 9(2):555–561
30. Picozzi VJ, Kozarek RA, Traverso LW (2003) Interferon-based adjuvant chemoradiation therapy after pancreaticoduodenectomy for pancreatic adenocarcinoma. Am J Surg 185(5):476–480

Chapter 9

The Role of Preoperative Biliary Decompression in Patients with Severe Malignant Obstructive Jaundice

Vincenzo Cangemi, Enrico Fiori

The advantage of preoperative biliary drainage (PBD) in severe and persistent obstructive jaundice, ensuing tumors of the head of the pancreas, of the Papilla of Vater or of the common bile duct, has been widely debated without achieving tangible or definitive results.

Attention has been focused in particular on the advisability or not of the use of biliary drainage as a preparatory phase of pancreaticoduodenectomy. In a 1999 editorial in Annals of Surgery, Lillimoe, discussed the problem in these terms: "To stent or not to stent, that is the question" [1].

The same problem is still debated today with the following recurring questions: (1) Is biliary drainage efficacious in the reduction of operative complications and mortality risk in patients with malignant obstructive jaundice? and (2) Is it burdened or not with inconveniences such as overweighing possible benefits or increasing complications or mortality after pancreatic resection procedures?

There are many, conflicting and inconclusive answers to these questions which have generated endless controversy. These answers may be summarized as follows: (1) biliary drainage is efficacious on the condition that it restores intestinal biliary flow [2–4]; (2) biliary drainage reduces morbidity, but does not reduce operative mortality [5, 6]; (3) biliary drainage reduces morbidity and operative mortality [3, 7, 8]; (4) biliary drainage is not efficacious, or if it is, it fails to compensate for its related inconveniences (biliary sepsis). It can be routinely used but only selectively [4, 9–13]; (5) biliary drainage is ineffective; it represents a risk factor and must be avoided [14–20]; (6) biliary drainage is efficacious if it is maintained at least 4-6 weeks prior to surgery [8, 21].

These different and conflicting opinions were collected among almost 40 out of the most important and significant publications available in the literature on that topic in a span of over two decades. Unfortunately, only 6 of these publications are pertinent to randomized studies [3, 8, 14, 22–24]. Moreover, two of these studies [22, 23] are barely reliable because they refer to external biliary drainage.

Some of these studies were recently selected by Sewnath [13] for a meta-analysis to point out that the use of drainage is justified only in select cases. This

A. Bolognese, L. Izzo (eds.), *Surgery in Multimodal Management of Solid Tumors.*
©Springer-Verlag Italia 2009

study has been criticized because of the excessive lack of uniformity of the studies deriving from single institutions. Therefore, no certainty has been provided by clinical research on the effective advantage of preoperative decompressive drainage in patients with severe malignant obstructive jaundice, eligible for pancreaticoduodenectomy, so that many surgeons, mainly Americans, have decided to no longer use this procedure.

In contrast, a contribution has been made by the huge number of experimental studies performed since 1970. Most of these support the use of PBD because it corrects or mitigates the damage due to obstructive jaundice: intestinal mucous barrier damage, functional and structural liver damage, immune system damage, macrophage activity of granulocytes and monocytes, nutritional damage, and damage to the intestinal collagen synthesis process [25–28].

Our experience regarding the use of PBD is the basis of a study carried out at the Department of Surgery "Pietro Valdoni" of the University of Rome. Seventy-eight patients with tumor of the head of the pancreas, of the Papilla of Vater or of the common bile duct and obstructive jaundice who underwent pancreaticoduodenectomy were included in this work.

Patients were subdivided into three groups. The first group of 21 patients showed bilirubin levels lower than 8.5 mg/100 mL and did not undergo biliary drainage. Of the 57 remaining patients whose bilirubin levels exceeded 8.5 mg/100 mL, 33 underwent internal or internal-external PBD, 2 were submitted to nasobiliary drainage (because of biliary sepsis), and 22 were not drained.

The 8.5 mg/100 mL blood bilirubin threshold was considered as a reference point between severe jaundice and less severe jaundice given the fact that such a threshold has been experimentally demonstrated to overlap with evident functional damage of the intestinal mucosa and with the translocation of germs and bacterial toxins from the intestinal lumen to the systemic portal circle. The consequence of bacterial and endotoxin translocation in the circle is an immediate systemic inflammatory response combined with a number of events that might lead to progressive multiple organ damage.

Drainage was maintained on average two weeks before surgery. Prophylactic broad-spectrum antibiotics were administered to drained patients immediately before and two days after drainage insertion. After surgery all patients received antibiotic treatment and total parenteral nutrition for 10 days.

Results

Complications ensuing from the drainage placement maneuver were observed in one patient only (perforation of the choledochus and moderate retroperitoneal biliary spreading). Clear signs of biliary infection were not observed in any of the drained patients. Operative complications and mortality are reported in Tables 9.1 and 9.2. In the drained patients with bilirubin levels exceeding 8.5 mg/100 mL operative mortality was 4.7% and morbidity 19.1%. In contrast, operative mortality and complications in undrained patients with bilirubin levels

Table 9.1 Operative complications: personal experience

	Bilirubinemia ≥8.5 mg/dL Drained		Undrained		Bilirubinemia <8.5 mg/dL Undrained		Total	
	No.	%	No.	%	No.	%	No.	%
Complications	7	20.0	10	45.4	4	19.1	21	6.9
Dehiscence of pancreaticojejunal anastomosis	2	5.7	2	9.1	1	4.7	5	6.4
Dehiscence of biliodigestive anastomosis	–	–	1	4.5	–	–	1	1.3
Biliodigestive fistula	1	2.8	–	–	–	–	1	1.3
Gastrointestinal bleeding	–	–	5	22.7*	–	–	5	6.4
Abdominal abscess	1	2.8	–	–	1	4.7	2	2.5
Renal failure	–	–	1	4.5	–	–	1	1.3
Others	2	5.7	1	4.5	1	4.7	4	5.1

*Fischer Test $p < 0.05$

Table 9.2 Operative mortality: personal experience

	Bilirubinemia ≥8.5 mg/dL Drained		Undrained		Bilirubinemia <8.5 mg/dL Undrained		Total	
	No.	%	No.	%	No.	%	No.	%
Mortality	2	5.7	3	13.6	1	4.7	6	7.6
Dehiscence of pancreaticojejunal anastomosis	2	5.7	1	4.5	1	4.7	4	5.1
Dehiscence of biliodigestive anastomosis	–	–	1	4.5	–	–	1	1.3
Renal failure	–	–	1	4.5	–	–	1	1.3

exceeding 8.5 mg/100 mL was 13.6 and 45.4% respectively, that is twice as high as the other groups of patients, even though this difference was not statistically significant.

In undrained patients with severe jaundice, gastrointestinal bleeding was observed in a higher percentage of cases, which was statistically significant (22.7% against 0). Renal insufficiency was shown in 4.5% of the undrained patients with bilirubin levels over 8.5 mg/100 mL and in none of the cases in the other groups. Anastomotic dehiscence and renal insufficiency represented the sole cause of death and were observed mainly in the groups of patients with bilirubin levels over 8.5 mg/100 mL who were not drained.

Discussion

The data emerging from our study outline that preoperative biliary drainage on the whole, but not significantly, reduces operative morbidity and mortality in patients with severe malignant obstructive jaundice after pancreaticoduodenectomy. Moreover, it reduces the risk of gastrointestinal bleeding significantly.

Our results suggest that PBD in patients with severe jaundice is efficacious, though its efficacy is restricted to the sole bleeding risk. We question whether this result might justify the routine use of PBD. Undoubtedly, experimental research encourages the routine use of PBD. In fact, there are strong pathophysiologic reasons supporting this attitude, which we believe appropriate to cite below.

The aggregation of bile salts leads to important structural mutations of the hepatic cells: cytoplasmic rarefaction with onset of vesicles, increase in the smooth plasmic reticulum and reduction of the rough reticulum, mitochondrial degeneration, cytoskeletal alterations and cell death in the most acute cases. These changes correspond with many important functional alterations: reduced activity of P 450 cytochrome, reduced detoxicant capability of drugs and toxic substances, reduced protein synthesis, reduced neoglycogenesis and ketogenesis, reduced glucose tolerability, reduced phagocytic activity of Küpffer cells and immune deficit [29, 30, 32–38].

The pathophysiologic mechanisms responsible for these modifications are not completely known. It is thought they might be due to an energy production deficit, to ATP and AMPc depletion, to an insufficiency of ATP-dependent "pumps", to the aggregation of calcium ions in the cytoplasm, to the damaging action of oxidant substances, to the tissue lipid perioxidation and the formation of arachidonic acid catabolites or to the toxic activity of thromboxane B2 [33].

More recent experimental studies have broadened the question about cholestatic hepatocyte damage, focusing attention on apoptotic cell mechanisms.

It has been demonstrated that the aggregation of bile salts acts on the Fas membrane receptor which activate the Fas-associated death domain (FADD) adaptor protein. FADD in turn recruits caspase-8, a protease that induces in turn the release of cathepsin B which is a cystein-protease. Cathepsin B, which is

activated by unspecified cytosolic substrates, induces the release of cytochrome
c from the mitochondria. Successively the activation of autocatalytic activation
of caspases occurs, causing the activation of endonucleasis and cytoskeletal
catabolism until the fragmentation of DNA and cell death with formation of
apoptotic bodies.

The Fas mechanism which enhances hepatocyte apoptosis is involved in the
local inflammatory response by inducing the release of inflammatory cytokines
(TNF-α) from the phagocyte cells. TNF-α and other cytokines are released by
Küpffer cells saturated with phagocytic bile. TNF-α also plays a leading role in
the apoptotic mechanisms. In fact, this cytokine acts on TNFR-1 tissue receptor
inducing the activation of small quantities of caspase-8, which are enough to
produce the release of lysosomal cathespin B. The subsequent shifts are comparable with those produced by the Fas mechanism [39–43].

The action of cytokines plays a leading role in the activation of the liver
inflammatory processes and through the stimulation of the stellate cells (or Ito
cells) it fosters the release of collagen and liver fibrogenesis with ensuing possible development of fibrosis.

From a systemic point of view the interruption of bile flow in the intestine
alters the barrier function of the intestinal mucosa making it permeable and
inducing the translocation of bacteria and their toxins in the portal circulation
and in the mesenteric lymphatic field and thereafter in the systemic circulation
and disguised as septicopyemic foci in different organs and tissues [23–26, 31,
44–47].

The process is facilitated by the immune deficit and by the incapacity of
Küpffer cells to perform a normal phagocyte function. The circulating bacterial
endotoxins activate macrophages and monocytes, activate endothelial cells fos-
tering the release of a great variability of pro-inflammatory mediators (TNF-α,
IL-1, IL-6, IL-8, NO, PAF), of O_2 free radicals, of endothelin and erythropoietin,
of arachidonic acid catabolites; furthermore they activate the complementary
system and the coagulation cascade originating a systemic inflammatory
response (SIRS, Systemic Inflammatory Response Syndrome). Lastly, the persistence or its amplification that might be caused by a second event or insult
(surgical trauma, septic foci) might foster a progressive multiple organ dysfunction (MODS, Multiple Organ Dysfunction Syndrome or MOF, Multiple Organ
Failure) [48–53].

The bile duct ligature in the rat causes an increase in TNF-α blood levels and
in the soluble receptors of TNF-α. Surgical trauma in the rat produces a further
massive increase in TNF-α and soluble receptors of TNF in blood. This increase
overlaps with a higher operative mortality.

The internal or internal-external biliary drainage that partially or totally re-
establishes the intestinal bile flow both in animals and humans decreases the levels of endotoxinemia and consequently the cytokine stimulus, reduces bacterial
translocation in the mesenteric lymph-nodes, corrects the immune deficit, recov-
ers the functional liver damage and the "clearance" functions of the liver phagocytic cells [12, 21, 25, 27, 33, 53–56]. In patients with jaundice with bilirubin

levels higher than 10 mg/100 mL the risk of postoperative bleeding complications is markedly increased [12]. Sepsis, renal insufficiency and bleeding gastritis are frequently observed in patients with jaundice who have undergone surgery and are easily correlated with endotoxinemia [55, 57–60].

Though these important, mostly experimental and pathophysiologic acquisitions favorably support PBD, there still remains the problem of whether its clinical use produces effective advantages or not.

The significant confusion about the systemic use of PBD in patients with malignant obstructive jaundice who are indicated for pancreaticoduodenectomy derives from the fact that a high risk of biliary infections, a more remarkable incidence of abdominal septic complications, and an inflammatory alteration against the main bile tract that might hinder biliodigestive anastomosis are imputable to PBD [61–63].

On the other hand, it is true that persistent obstructive jaundice is itself a risk factor for biliary infection. Moreover some recent studies have outlined that the presence of the bacteriophila frequently observed after drainage is not as much linked to the drainage itself as to the rather rough endoscopic maneuvers of stent insertion. Other investigators report an evident correlation among biliary sepsis ensuing drainage and the postoperative abdominal septic complications [61–64].

Some experimental and clinical studies have shown that the benefits of PBD in terms of recovery of the damage caused by cholestasis become evident 6 weeks after the drainage insertion [65, 66]. These findings are the result of the following question: is it legitimate to delay pancreatic resection for 6 weeks in favor of potential but still unconfirmed advantages when we are dealing with malignant disease which is usually very aggressive? Taking into consideration the different trends, it emerges that in a span of more than three decades of studies and research on this topic, at present we tend to believe, in agreement with other investigators, that the use of drainage must not be prejudicially avoided, but rather it must be used selectively.

The following indications might prove reasonably effective: undernourished patients with high risk of sepsis, patients with blood coagulation disorders or disease associated with high bleeding risk, patients with liver or renal failure and of course patients who require neoadjuvant chemotherapeutic treatment.

References

1. Lillemoe KD (1999) Preoperative biliary drainage and surgical outcome. Ann Surg 230:143–144
2. Gouma DJ, Moody G (1984) Preoperative percutaneous drainage: use or abuse. Surg Gastroenterol 3:74–80
3. Smith RC, Pooley M, George CRP et al (1985) Preoperative percutaneous transhepatic internal drainage in obstructive jaundice: a randomized controlled trial examining renal function. Surgery 97:641–647
4. Naakeb A, Pitt HA (1995) The role of preoperative biliary decompression in obstructive jaundice. Hepatogastroenterology 42:332–337
5. Denning DA, Ellison EC, Carey LC (1981) Preoperative percutaneous transhepatic biliary

decompression operative morbidity in patients with obstructive jaundice. Am J Surg 141:61–65

6. Lygidakis NJ, Van der Heyde MN, Lubbers MJ (1987) Evaluation of preoperative biliary drainage in the surgical management of pancreatic head carcinoma. Acta Chir Scand 153:665–668

7. Gundry SR, Strodel WE, Knol JA et al (1984) Efficacy of preoperative biliary tract decompression in patients with ostructive jaundice. Arch Surg 119:703–708

8. Wig JD, Kumar H, Suri S et al (1999) Usefulness of percutaneous transhepatic biliary drainage in patients with surgical jaundice – a prospective randomised study. J Assoc Physicians India 47:271–274

9. Marcus SG, Dobriansky M, Shamamian P et al (1998) Endoscopic biliary drainage before pancreaticoduodenectomy for periampullary malignancies. J Clin Gastroenterol 26:125–129

10. Sohn TA, Yeo CJ, Cameron JL et al (2000) Do preoperative biliary stents increase postpancreaticoduodenectomy complications? J Gastrointest Surg 4:258–267

11. Sewnath ME, Birjmohun RS, Rauws EA et al (2001) The effect of preoperative biliary drainage on postoperative complications after pancreaticoduodenectomy. Am Coll Surg 192:726–734

12. Srivastava S, Sikora SS, Kumar A et al (2001) Outcome following pancreaticoduodenectomy in patients undergoing preoperative biliary drainage. Dig Surg 18:381–387

13. Sewnath ME, Karsten TM, Prins MH et al (2002) A meta-analysis on the efficacy of preoperative biliary drainage for tumors causing obstructive jaundice. Ann Surg 236:17–27

14. Lai EC, Chu KM, Lo CY et al (1992) Surgery for malignant obstructive jaundice: analysis of mortality. Surgery 112:891–896

15. Karsten TM, Allema JH, Reinders M et al (1996) Preoperative biliary drainage, colonisation of bile and postoperative complications in patients with tumours of the pancreatic head: a retrospective analysis of 241 consecutive patients. Eur J Surg 162:881–888

16. Heslin MJ, Brooks AD, Hochwald SN et al (1998) A preoperative biliary stent in associated with increased complications after pancreatoduodenectomy. Arch Surg 133:149–154

17. Povoski SP, Karpeh MS Jr, Conlon KC et al (1999) Association of preoperative biliary drainage with postoperative outcome following pancreaticoduodenectomy. Ann Surg 230:131–142

18. Martignoni ME, Wagner M, Krähenbühl L et al (2001) Effect of preoperative biliary drainage on surgical outcome after pancreatoduodenectomy. Am J Surg 181:52–59

19. Pisters PWT, Hudec WA, Hess KR et al (2001) Effect of preoperative biliary decompression on pancreaticoduodenectomy-associated morbidity in 300 consecutive patients. Ann Surg 234:47–55

20. Kahl S, Zimmermann S, Pross M et al (2003) Endoscopic biliary in patients with pancreatic cancer. Zentralbl Chir 128:406–410

21. Watanapa P (1996) Recovery patterns of liver function after complete and partial surgical biliary decompression. Am J Surg 171:230–235

22. Hatfield ARW, Tobias R, Terblanche J et al (1982) Preoperative external biliary drainage in obstructive jaundice:a prospective controlled clinical trial. Lancet 2:896–899

23. Mc Pherson GAD, Benjamin IS, Hodgson HJF et al (1984) Preoperative percutaneous transhepatic biliary drainage: the results of a controlled trial. Br J Surg 71:371–375

24. Pitt HA, Gomes AS, Lois JF et al (1985) Does percutaneous biliary drainage reduce operative risk or increase hospital cost? Ann Surg 201:545–553

25. Rougheen PT, Gouma DJ, Kulkarni AD et al (1986) Impaired specific cell-mediated immunity in experimental biliary obstruction and its reversibility by internal biliary drainage. J Surg Res 41:113–125

26. Gouma DJ, Coelho JCU, Fisher JD et al (1986) Endotoxemia after of biliary obstruction by internal and external drainage in rats. Am J Surg 151:476–479

27. Gouma DJ, Julio CU, Coelho PD et al (1986) The effect of preoperative internal and external biliary drainage on mortality of jaundiced rats. Arch Surg 122:731–4

28. Parks RW, Halliday MI, McCrory DC et al. (2003) Host immune responses and intestinal

permeability in patients with jaundice. Br J Surg 90:239–245
29. Thompson RL, Hoper M, Diamond T et al (1990) Development and reversibility of T lymphocyte dysfunction in experimental obstructive jaundice. Br J Surg 77:1229–1232
30. Shibatani N, Yamamoto S, Kubota Y et al (2002) Neutrophil chemotaxis in bile duct-obstructed rats, and effect of internal biliary drainage. Hepatogastroenterology 49:918–923
31. Bailey ME (1986) Endotoxin bile salys and renal function in obstructive jaundice. Br J Surg 63:774–778
32. Schaffner F, Bacchin P, Hutterer F et al (1986) Mechanism of cholestasis: structural and biochemical changes in the liver and serum in rats after bile duct ligation. Gastroenterology 60:888–897
33. Ido M, Higashiguchi T, Tanigawa K et al (1995) Cell biological evaluation of biliary drainage prior to hepatectomy in obstructive jaundice. Hepatogastroenterology 42:308–316
34. Regan MC, Keane RM, Little D et al (1994) Postoperative immunological function and jaundice. Br J Surg 81:271–273
35. Megison SM, Dunn CW, Horton JW et al (1991) Effects of relief of biliary obstruction on mononuclear phagocyte system function and cell mediated immunity. Br J Surg 78:568–571
36. Ozawa K, Takasan H, Kitamura D et al (1973) Alteration of liver mitochondrial in a patients with biliary obstruction due to liver carcinoma. Am J Surg 126:653–657
37. Cainzos M, Potel J, Puente JL (1988). Anergy in jaundiced patients. Br J Surg 75:147–149
38. Koyama K, Takagi Y, Ito K et al (1981) Experimental and clinical studies on the effect of biliary drainage in obstructive jaundice. Am J Surg 142:293–299
39. Faouzi S, Burckhardt BE, Hanson JC et al (2001) Anti-Fas induces hepatic chemokines and promotes inflammation by an NF-kB-independent, caspase-3-dependent Pathway. J Biol Chem 276:49077–49082
40. Guicciardi ME, Deussing J, Miyoshi H et al (2000) Cathepsin B contributes to TNF-a-mediated hepatocyte apoptosis by promoting mitochondrial release of cytochrome c. J Clin Invest 106:1127–137
41. Murphy FR, Issa R, Zhou X et al (2002) Inibition of apoptosis of activated hepatic stellate cells by tissue inhibitor of metalloproteinase-1 is mediated via effects on matrix metalloproteinase inhibition. J Biol Chem 277:11069–11076
42. Canbay A, Guicciardi ME, Higuchi H et al (2003) Cathepsin B inactivation attenuates hepatic injury and fibrosis during cholestasis. J Clin Invest 112:152–159
43. Faubion WA, Guicciardi ME, Miyoshi H et al (1999) Toxic bile salts induce rodent hepatocyte apoptosis via direct activation of Fas. J Clin Invest 103:137–145
44. Slocum MM, Sittig KM, Specian RD et al (1992) Absence of intestinal bile promotes bacterial translocation. Am Surg 58:305–310
45. Diamond T, Dolan S, Thompson RLE et al (1990) Development and reversal of endotoxemia and endotoxin-related death in obstructive jaundice. Surgery 108:370-375
46. Clements WDB, Parks R, Erwin P et al (1996) Role of the gut in the pathophysiology of extrahepatic biliary obstruction. Gut 39:587–593
47. Ding JW, Andersson R, Soltesz V et al (1993) The role of bile and bile acids in bacterial translocation in obstructive jaundice in rats. Eur Surg Res 25:11–19
48. Ballinger AB, Wolley JA, Ahmed M et al (1998) Persistent systemic inflammatory response after stent insertion in patients with malignant bile duct obstruction. Gut 42:555–559
49. Glauser MP, Zanetti G, Baumgartner JD et al (1992) Lo shock settico: patogenesi. Lancet 9:258–266
50. Padillo FJ, Muntane J, Montero JL et al (2002) Effect of internal biliary drainage on plasma levels of endotoxin, cytokines, and c–reactive protein in patients with obstructive jaundice. World J Surg 26:1328–1332
51. Giacometti A, Cirioni O, Ghiselli R et al (2003) Administration of protegrin peptide IB-367 to prevent endotoxin induced mortality in bile duct ligated rats. Gut 52:874–878
52. Fahey TJ, Yoshioka T, Shires T et al (1996) The role of tumour necrosis factor and nitric oxide in the acute cardiovascular response to endotoxin. Ann Surg 223:63–69
53. Kimmings AN, van Deventer SJH, Obertop H et al (2000) Endotoxin, cytokines, and endo-

toxin binding proteins in obstructive jaundice and after preoperative biliary drainage. Gut 46:725–731

54. Ding JW, Andersson R, Soltesz V et al (1993) The effect of biliary decompression on bacterial translocation in jaundiced rats. HPB Surg 7:99–110

55. Ding JW, Andersson R, Stenram U et al (1992). Effect of biliary decompression on reticuloendothelial function in jaundiced rats. Br J Surg 79:648–652

56. Grewe JW, Maessen JG, Tiebosch T (1990) Prevention of postoperative complications in jaundice rats: internal biliary drainage versus oral lactulose. Ann Surg 212:221–227

57. Dixon JM, Armstrong CP, Davies GC (1984) Pre-operative biliary drainage. Br J Surg 71:1007

58. Wilkinson SP, Moodie H, Stomatakis JG (1976) Endotoxaemia and renal failure in cirrhosis and obstructive jaundice. Br Med J 2:1415–1418

59. Cahill CJ (1983) Prevention of postoperative renal failure in patients with obstructive jaundice. The role of bile salts. Br J Surg 70:590–595

60. Cahill CJ, Pain JA, Bailey ME (1987) Bile salts, endotoxin and renal function in obstructive jaundice. Surg Gynecol Obstet 165:519–522

61. Aly EA, Johnson CD (2001) Preoperative biliary drainage before resection in obstructive jaundice. Dig Surg 18:84–89

62. Povoski SP, Karpeh MS, Conlon KC et al (1999) Preoperative biliary drainage: impact on intraoperative bile culture and infectious morbidity and mortality after pancreaticoduodenectomy. J Gastrointest Surg 3:496–505

63. Hochwald SN, Burke EC, Jarnagin WR et al (1999) Association of preoperative biliary stenting with increased postoperative infectious complications in proximal cholangiocarcinoma. Arch Surg 134:261–266

64. Coppola R, Riccioni ME, Ciletti S et al (2001) Periampullary tumors. Analysis of 319 consecutive cases submitted to preoperative endoscopic biliary drainage. Surg Endosc 15:1135–9

65. Fiori E, Atella F, Gazzanelli S et al (1994) The usefulness of biliary drainage for restoring liver function in obstructive jaundice. Panminerva Medica 36:171–178

66 Fiori E, Macchiarelli G, Schillaci A et al (2003) Hepatocyte ultrastructural aspects after preoperative biliary drainage in pancreatic cancer patients with cholestatic jaundice. Anticancer Res 23:4859–4863

Chapter 10

Surgery in Multimodal Treatment of Cancer: Peritoneal Carcinomatosis

Angelo Di Giorgio, Fabio Accarpio, Simone Sibio, Daniele Biacchi, Sergio Gazzanelli, Anna M. Baccheschi, Tommaso Cornali, Marisa Di Seri, Linda Cerbone, Paolo Sammartino

Until recent years a diagnosis of peritoneal carcinomatosis (PC) from intra-abdominal solid tumors carried a uniformly fatal prognosis, often within weeks or months. Since the 1980s, following the intuition of an American surgeon, Paul Sugarbaker, combined treatment modalities of PC have developed considerably. Since the first pioneering approaches on the treatment of "pseudomyxoma peritonei" [1], interest has grown particularly in recent years among the international scientific community regarding the combined treatment (cytoreductive surgery plus perioperative intraperitoneal chemotherapy) of peritoneal surface malignancy (PSM).

Currently about fifty institutions in the world, located mainly in the United States and Western Europe, treat these patients according to therapeutic criteria that have undergone a slow but constant process of homogeneity both due to the institution in 1998 of bi-annual international workshops and to an internet web site (www.peritonectomy.com) in which experts exchange experience and information on current research.

However, much remains to be done. In fact, despite significant improvements in disease-free and overall survival having been demonstrated in patients with PC of appendiceal, colorectal and ovarian cancers and with diffuse malignant peritoneal mesothelioma, [2–5] it still appears that a minority of patients with peritoneal spread are approached in this manner and too often these patients are judged untreatable, and therefore denied the possibility of cure [6].

Nonetheless, a recurrent problem is the fact that these patients come before the surgeon as a last resort after the failure of multiple chemotherapy lines. As a result they are not ideal surgical candidates due to malnutrition, poor performance status and usually intractable ascites. Many questions remain that still need to be addressed via further studies, and greater cooperation between oncologists and surgeons is required so that these combined treatment modalities of cytoreductive surgery (CRS) and perioperative intraperitoneal chemotherapy (PIC) can become a part of "standard care" for patients with PSM.

A. Bolognese, L. Izzo (eds.), *Surgery in Multimodal Management of Solid Tumors.*
©Springer-Verlag Italia 2009

Rationale

Surgery for cancer has evolved from the treatment of primary malignancy to include the management of metastatic disease. In the setting of gastrointestinal cancer, early success with this new concept occurred with surgery of locally recurrent colon and rectal cancer, and this was followed by the benefits achieved in the resection of liver metastases from large bowel malignancy in a selected group of patients [7]. Extension of the concept of complete surgical eradication of metastatic disease to bring about long-term survival to selected patients with PSM has been pioneered by Paul Sugarbaker [8]. Since the mid 1990s significant efforts have been made to improve the outcome of patients with PSM and currently CRS and PIC are gaining recognition as treatment options for a variety of peritoneal surface-based malignancies.

Successful management of PSM requires a combined approach that utilizes CRS (peritonectomy procedures) and PIC. Peritonectomy procedures are used in the area of visible cancer nodules in an attempt to leave the patients with only microscopic residual disease. Both visceral and parietal peritonectomy are necessary for complete cytoreduction which is essential if the treatment is to produce long-term survival. Between one and six peritonectomy procedures may be required [9–11] and their utilization depends on the distribution, volume and depth of invasion of the malignancy disseminated within the peritoneal space.

The "tumour cell entrapment" hypothesis explains the lack of long-term benefit in patients who undergo treatment of PSM using surgery alone. This theory relates through a multiple-step process, starting by free intraperitoneal tumor emboli, which are then entrapped by the fibrin in the traumatized tissue surface and successively grow in the wound-healing process. This phenomenon may cause a high incidence of surgical treatment failure in patients treated only by cytoreduction unless PIC is used.

PIC is performed either during the procedure or early in the postoperative setting, in all cases before adhesion creates multiple barriers to free fluid access. For the chemotherapy solution, high molecular weight cytotoxic drugs are used that allow lengthy exposure of the peritoneal surface to pharmacologically active molecules with limited systemic effects. Early studies in the literature describe early postoperative intraperitoneal chemotherapy (EPIC) being used for four to five days after surgery. In recent years intraperitoneal chemotherapy has been demonstrated to be potentiated by hyperthermia, and hyperthermic intraperitoneal chemotherapy (HIPEC) is currently in use [12].

Selection Criteria and Treatment Results

To balance the risk and benefits of these procedures knowledgeable patient selection is mandatory. In the current literature the overall mortality associated with CRS and HIPEC differs from 1 to 10% and morbidity ranges from 20 to 50% [13].

The adoption of strict selection criteria is a key element in limiting complication rates and improving outcome in these patients. The eligibility requirements for treatment in the current literature are as follows: histologically confirmed diagnosis of PSM; age ≤75 years; no extra-abdominal metastases; performance status 0–2 according to WHO criteria and adequate cardiac, renal, hepatic, and bone marrow function [14].

The intra-abdominal extension of the disease and the criteria used to evaluate it are fundamental issues. The extent of PC was usually recorded according to the Peritoneal Cancer Index (PCI) proposed by Sugarbaker [15]. The PCI is a clinical summary of the size of intraperitoneal nodules and the distribution of PSM. The number of nodules is not scored, only the size of the largest one. In order to assess the distribution of peritoneal surface disease the abdominopelvic regions are utilized. For each of these 13 regions a lesion score is determined; the summation of the lesion score in each of the 13 abdominopelvic regions is the PCI for that patient. A maximal score is 39 (13 x 3) (Fig. 10.1).

Because patients with extensive carcinomatosis generally have a poor prognosis and may have severe postoperative complications, current consensus recommends that candidates for surgery (e.g. in colorectal carcinomatosis) should be strictly selected according to the PCI, using a PCI score around 15 to 20 as an ideal threshold value [16, 17].

Even though correctly identifying the spread of PC remains an intraoperative task, by integrating the preoperative clinical and imaging findings, the likelihood

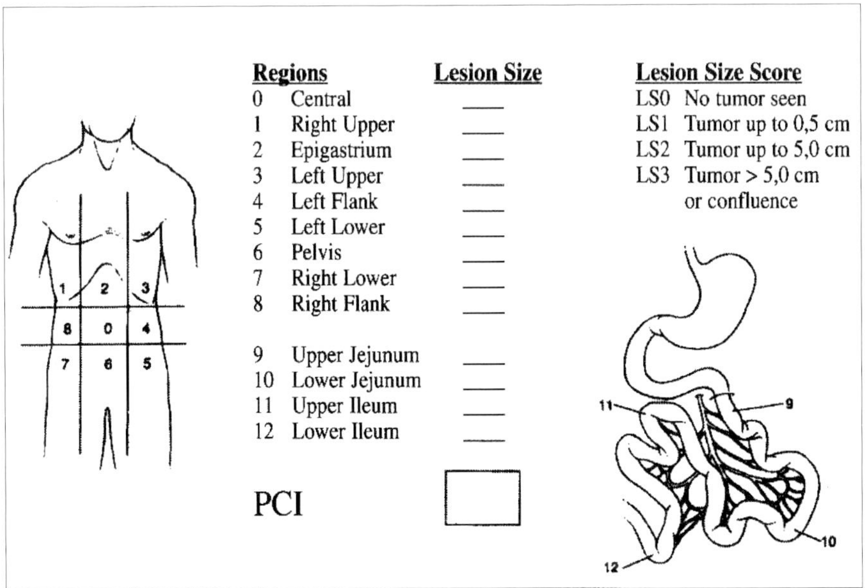

Fig. 10.1 Peritoneal Cancer Index

of achieving satisfactory cytoreduction can be reliably predicted. The judicious indication of the different methodologies (CT, MRI, PET, laparoscopy) in the preoperative work up should aid the careful selection of patients according to the PCI score, establish the surgical strategy for the cytoreduction, and finally estimate prognosis and the risk of morbidity and mortality related to the treatment [18]. The empiric values of these predictive systems nonetheless stress the need to maintain the difficult balance between unnecessary exploration and inappropriate non exploration.

The main prognostic factor in patients with PSM is the level of cytoreduction obtained. This issue is evaluated according to the Completeness of Cytoreduction Score (CCS) proposed by Sugarbaker [8] as follows: CC0 no residual disease; CC1 residual nodules measuring less than 2.5 mm; CC2 nodules measuring between 2.5 mm and 2.5 cm and CC3 residual nodules greater than 2.5 cm.

The long-term results of the treatment of PSM show how survival is related to the tumor which caused PC (and often to its specific histologic features), to the diffusion of intra-abdominal disease (PCI) and to the level of cytoreduction obtained (CCS).

Pseudomyxoma peritonei from appendicular tumors was the first diffuse peritoneal tumor historically treated due to the specificity of its natural history with slow growth, low aggressivity with production of large quantities of mucin through which the tumor cells colonize the peritoneal spaces with scarce tendency towards diffusion by lymphatic and hematogenous pathways. In pseudomyxoma the histologic features show a determinant prognostic role as demonstrated by the different survival results between diffuse peritoneal adenomucinosis (DPAM) and peritoneal mucinous carcinomatosis (PMCA), the latter resembling other carcinomatoses of colorectal origin [19].

Similarly a recent report about the treatment of peritoneal mesothelioma suggests that the nuclear size of the tumor cells is the main significant prognostic element in a multivariate analysis suggesting classification based exclusively on this parameter [5].

The results of treatment of PC from ovarian or colorectal cancer appear to be much less influenced by specific histologic features and much more by clinical parameters such as PCI and CCS. Although transcelomic diffusion of ovarian cancer is such a typical feature of this tumor, the combined treatment modalities (CRS plus PIC) found favor later than in other carcinomatoses. This was due to the high chemotherapy-sensitivity of ovarian cancer and to the early good response obtained by adjuvant platinum and taxane regimens. Although this therapy initially seems effective, about half of the patients relapse within 5 years and the high incidence of peritoneal recurrence calls for the adoption of integrated treatment (CRS plus PIC) in ovarian carcinomatosis according to the standard criteria adopted for other PSM [20, 21]. The analysis of survival results in ovarian carcinomatosis shows that the volume of peritoneal disease (PCI) has a less significant impact with respect to the level of the cytoreduction obtained (CCS), the latter being the only significant prognostic factor when a multivariate statistical analysis has been carried out [4].

Finally, colorectal carcinomatosis has been to date the subject with the greatest amount of data available and the treatment results of hundreds of cases have been published [3, 22]. In selected cases when complete cytoreduction has been obtained, survival reaches over 40% at 5 years, an inconceivable result only a few years ago [23]. Furthermore, the only randomized study comparing the combined approach (CRS plus PIC) versus systemic chemotherapy was carried out on these patients [24]. The results of this study were so different and in favor of the combined approach that the trial was stopped for ethical reasons. Unlike ovarian carcinomatosis in colorectal carcinomatosis the volume of peritoneal diseases (PCI) is a limiting factor in achieving optimal cytoreduction and in the final analysis in patient prognosis. As previously stated, an ideal selection should identify candidates for surgery among patients with a PCI between 15 and 20. Recently the guidelines in the treatment of colorectal carcinomatosis have been reported in a Consensus Statement that involved more than 70 surgeons and 55 international treatment centers throughout the world, thus opening the way to substantial acceptance of the combined approach (CRS plus PIC) as the gold standard in the treatment of this disease [25].

Patients and Methods

From November 2000 to April 2008 an open prospective single-center nonrandomized phase 2 study was conducted at the Department of Surgery "Pietro Valdoni". Patients presenting resectable PC from gastrointestinal gynecological or mesothelial origin were considered eligible.

The inclusion criteria were age younger than 75 years; a histologically or cytologically confirmed diagnosis; performance status 0–2 (WHO); adequate cardiac, renal, hepatic, and bone marrow function; resectable disease; and informed written consent. The exclusion criteria were extra-abdominal metastases; other malignancies except breast cancer; unresectable disease; and active infections or severe associated medical conditions.

The pretreatment evaluation comprised a complete medical history and physical examination, as well as laboratory investigations including blood counts, blood coagulation tests, renal and liver-function tests, and tumor markers. Diagnostic imaging including multislice spiral computed tomography (CT) or abdominopelvic magnetic resonance imaging (MRI) or both, bone scintigraphy and in patients with predominant recurrent disease, positron emission tomography (PET) scan.

Disease was defined as resectable if from the patient's history and findings on diagnostic imaging the surgeon judged it possible to obtain satisfactory surgical cytoreduction to slow or arrest the natural history of the disease. The treatment plan envisaged extensive surgical cytoreduction aimed at removing all visible disease plus immediate HIPEC and adjuvant systemic chemotherapy starting at least six weeks after discharge according to the patient's general status. The study protocol was approved by the medical ethics committee of the hospital.

Surgical Procedure (Peritonectomy)

Patients were placed in a low lithotomy position; the abdomen was carefully explored through a midline incision from the xiphoid process to the pubic symphysis and a self-retaining retractor was positioned. At laparotomy the extent of peritoneal carcinomatosis was recorded according to the PCI. Aggressive surgical cytoreduction was then undertaken to leave the patient with no visible disease. Visceral and parietal peritoneal resection is the basis of peritonectomy procedures. One or more peritonectomy procedures were required depending on the distribution and volume of peritoneal carcinomatosis. Parietal peritoneal resection entailed total or partial removal of the pelvic peritoneum, the abdominal wall peritoneum, the diaphragmatic peritoneum, the greater and lesser omentum and the peritoneum of the bursa omentalis. Small numbers of scattered peritoneal implants were resected or ablated with high-voltage electrocautery, radiofrequency technology (TissueLink BPS 6.0) or an argon beam coagulator. Bulky disease such as confluent implants involving an extensive area was usually removed with one of the major peritonectomy procedures. In all patients, pelvic carcinomatosis was managed with pelvic peritonectomy and anterior parietal peritonectomy below the umbilical transverse line. Visceral resection envisaged resection of all organs or structures involved by primary tumor or metastatic implants. When visceral resection proved impossible or when nodules were small or isolated, we resected or ablated the nodules using the aforementioned techniques. As for disease setting, primary cytoreduction was classified as the treatments of PC performed together with the resection of the primary tumor, whereas secondary cytoreduction was classified as the treatment of metachronous carcinomatosis. All surgical procedures were recorded, as were the number and type of resections and other reconstructive procedures. The completeness of cytoreduction (CC) was scored as proposed by Sugarbaker.

Hyperthermic Intraperitoneal Chemotherapy (HIPEC)

At the end of each surgical procedure, HIPEC was given under general anesthesia with the closed technique and during hemodynamic monitoring. Four drains were positioned for HIPEC inflow/outflow and temperature monitoring; two drains (27 F) placed under the right and left diaphragmatic cupola for inflow, one drain (30 F) was inserted into the pelvis for outflow and the last drain (24 F) was placed near the first jejunal loop as a peritoneal thermal probe. The abdominal wall was then definitively and completely closed with a single watertight absorbable continuous suture. Two further thermal probes were positioned for temperature monitoring, outside the abdominal wall at the inflow and outflow drains and another pharyngoesophageal temperature probe was inserted to measure core temperature.

The inflow/outflow drains were connected to a closed extracorporeal sterile circuit in which a 2 to 4 l perfusate was circulated by means of a peristaltic pump at a flow rate of 500 mL/min. The closed sterile circuit was heated by means of a thermal exchanger connected to the heating circuit (EXIPER, Euromedical, Italy).

When peritoneal and outflow temperatures reached a thermal plateau of 41°C (generally within 10-15 minutes), HIPEC at inflow temperatures ranging from 45 to 46°C was given for 60 minutes with cisplatin at a dose of 75 mg/m²/l (for ovarian carcinomatosis), oxaliplatin at a dose of 460 mg/m²/l (for colonic and gastric carcinomatosis) and cisplatin at a dose of 25 mg/m²/l + doxorubicin at a dose of 7 mg/m²/l (for peritoneal mesothelioma) under close monitoring of respiratory and hemodynamic variables. Trendelenburg/anti-Trendelenburg and laterolateral inclinations of the recumbent patient were changed every five minutes to guarantee that the entire peritoneal surface was perfused. During perfusion, the intra- and extra-abdominal temperatures were recorded every five minutes. After the procedure the abdomen was washed with 3–4 l of sterile saline at 37°C.

Morbidity and Toxicity

During the immediate postoperative period patients were assisted in an intensive care unit (ICU) for at least 24 hours; each patient was carefully monitored for potential complications or symptoms or both, related or unrelated to combined surgery and HIPEC. Pharmacologic toxicity was scored using the WHO toxicity grading scale for chemotherapy [26]. Treatment-related morbidity and mortality were classified as grade I: no complication, grade II: minor complications, grade III: major complications requiring re-operation, ICU admission or interventional radiology, and grade IV: in-hospital mortality [27].

Follow-up

After hospital discharge, patients were referred to the medical oncologist to plan systemic chemotherapy. Patients were followed up every six months with abdominal CT scan, positron emission tomography (PET SCAN), measurement of serum markers, complete blood cell count, blood chemical analysis including liver and renal function tests and any further evaluation indicated by the patients' clinical presentation.

Survival and Statistical Analysis

Differences between groups of observations were analyzed by a chi-square test. The Kaplan-Meier method was used to construct survival curves and a log rank test was used to assess the significance of the difference between curves. The Cox regression model was used to determine the prognostic value of independent variables. p-values <0.05 were considered statistically significant. The NCSS (Kaysville, Utah) package was used to analyze the dataset and perform statistical tests.

Results

Patients

Eighty patients with a median age of 61.1 years (range 32–75) with PC from different sites of origin were prospectively enrolled in the study from November 2000 to April 2008. Seven more patients initially enrolled underwent a palliative procedure alone and are not considered in this report. Of the 80 patients treated, 54 were affected by ovarian carcinomatosis and 26 by carcinomatosis from other primary malignancy. Thirty-nine patients were treated as primary cytoreduction, and the other 41 underwent secondary cytoreduction. All 41 patients undergoing secondary cytoreduction had already undergone one or more operations for the primary cancer (range 1–4 laparotomies) plus chemotherapy (range 1-3 lines). Patient characteristics are summarized in Table 10.1.

Surgical procedure

The mean PCI calculated according to Sugarbaker criteria was 15.1 (range 6–35) for ovarian carcinomatosis and 19.6 (range 5–39) for the other group. Overall the 80 patients treated required a total of 458 surgical procedures; mean 6.3 (range 4-10) for ovarian carcinomatosis and 4.5 (range 1–7) in other cases (Table 10.2). In 68 of 80 patients (85%) debulking achieved optimal cytoreduction (scored CC0 or CC1), whereas in 12 patients (15%) it left macroscopic residual disease (scored CC2 or CC3). In all but one patient who had a low PCI (less than or equal to the mean value of each group) debulking achieved complete cytoreduction, whereas in patients with a higher PCI (greater than the mean value) debulking achieved optimal cytoreduction in 70% of cases (chi-square test: p <0.0002 for ovarian carcinomatosis, p <0.007 for others) (Table 10.3). All variables regarding surgical outcomes including the duration of the operative procedures, the mean blood loss, the mean number of blood and plasma units transfused together with the mean ICU stay and the mean hospital stay are summarized in Table 10.4.

Hyperthermic Intraperitoneal Chemotherapy (HIPEC)

Of the total 80 patients in the series, 77 underwent HIPEC at the end of surgery. Three patients did not undergo HIPEC owing to their unstable postoperative hemodynamic conditions and instead underwent a 5-day course of postoperative intraperitoneal unheated chemotherapy after ICU discharge. The mean time to reach a temperature higher than 40°C in the abdominal cavity was 10 minutes and the intraperitoneal temperature invariably remained over 41°C and mainly over 42°C (mean, 42.7°C, range, 41.0–43.3°C). None of the HIPEC procedures

Table 10.1 Patient demographic and clinical characteristics (80 patients)

Variables	Ovary (54)	Other (26)
Age (years)	Mean (range)	Mean (range)
	60.6 (32–75)	62 (35–75)
Disease setting	No. (%)	No. (%)
– Primary cytoreduction	26 (48.1)	13 (50)
– Secondary cytoreduction	28 (51.9)	13 (50)
Previous chemotherapy	No. (%)	No. (%)
– No	21 (38.8)	12 (46.2)
– Yes	33 (61.2)	14 (53.8)
– Neoadjuvant	6	0
– Adjuvant	27	13
Performance status (WHO)	No. (%)	No. (%)
– 0	23 (42.6)	9 (34.6)
– 1	15 (27.8)	12 (46.1)
– 2	16 (29.6)	5 (19.3)
Intestinal obstruction	No. (%)	No. (%)
– Absent	38 (70.4)	16 (61.5)
– Present	16 (29.6)	10 (39.5)
Ascites	No. (%)	No. (%)
– Absent	23 (42.6)	10 (38.5)
– Present	31 (57.4)	16 (61.5)
Comorbidity	No. (%)	No. (%)
– Absent	41 (75.9)	20 (76.9)
– Present	13 (24.1)	6 (23.1)
Ca125 level (U/mL)	Mean	
	577.4 (12–6800)	
Origin	No. (%)	No. (%)
– Ovary	54 (67.5)	
– Colon		9 (11.2)
– Stomach		5 (6.2)
– Appendix		1 (1.2)
– Breast		3 (3.8)
– Primary unknown		2 (2.5)
– Mesothelioma		3 (3.8)
– Sarcoma		3 (3.8)

Table 10.2 Surgical treatment

Type of resection	Ovary			Other		
	Primary (No.)	Secondary (No.)	Total (No.)	Primary (No.)	Secondary (No.)	Total (No.)
Hysterectomy +/ adnexectomy	26	6	32	5	3	8-
Pelvic mass resection		8	8		1	1
Omental resection	25	20	45	11	8	19
Intestinal resection						
– Colorectal resection		4	21	3	3	6
– Total colectomy/rectal resection	17	11	16	4	1	5
– Other colic resection	5	4	7	3	5	8
– Appendicectomy	3	3	15	4	2	6
– Small bowel resection	12	9	15	5	9	14
– Gastric resection	6	1	1	1	1	2
Splenectomy	7	13	20	5	3	8
Cholecystectomy	5	8	13	3	1	4
Liver resection	1	2	3			
Total cystectomy	1		1			
Bladder resection	1	2	3		1	1
Total peritonectomy	4	6	10	3	1	4
Partial peritonectomy	20	17	37	6	3	9
Abdominal wall resection	3	4	7	1	3	4
Resection or reduction cancer implants	14	26	40	7	7	14
Paraortic and pelvic lymphadenectomy	22	8	30	1		1
Lymphadenectomy in 9 other sites	7	16	1		1	
By-pass					3	3
Total	181	159	340	63	55	118
Mean number of procedures	7 (4–10)	5.7 (4–9)	6.3 (4–10)	4.8 (1–6)	4.2 (1–7)	4.5 (1–7)

Table 10.3 Impact of peritoneal cancer index (*PCI*) on completeness of cytoreduction (*CC score*)

Ovary CC score	PCI ≤15 No. cases (%)	PCI >15 No. cases (%)	Other CC score	PCI ≤20 No. cases (%)	PCI >20 No. cases (%)
0	27 (93.1)	10 (40)	0	12 (85.8)	2 (16.7)
1	2 (6.9)	10 (40)	1	1 (7.1)	4 (33.3)
2	0	3 (12)	2	1 (7.1)	3 (25)
3	0	2 (8)	3	0	3 (25)
Total	29	25	Total	14	12

Mean PCI: 15.1 (6–35)
Chi-square test: $p = 0.0002$

Mean PCI: 19.6 (8–39)
Chi-square test: $p = 0.007$

Table 10.4 Surgical outcome

Ovary	Other
Duration procedure (min)	522 (180–780)	492 (180–840)
– Primary cytoreduction	506 (300–780)	534 (180–840)
– Secondary cytoreduction	477 (180–720)	445 (180–720)
Blood loss (mL)	1499 (100–4900)	2414 (0–30000)
– Primary cytoreduction	1662 (400–4900)	3588 (0–30000)
– Secondary cytoreduction	1353 (100–3100)	1141 (400–2500)
Blood transfusion (units)	3.5 (0–8)	4.6 (0–25)
Plasma transfusion (units)	5.2 (0–10)	5 (0–16)
ICU stay (h)	49.3 (0–480)	96.5 (12–1440)

Morbidity	Ovary No. (%)	Other No. (%)	Complications (No.)	Treatment
– Grade 1	30 (55.5)	18 (69.2)		
– Grade 2	10 (18.5)	3 (11.5)	pleural effusion (4)	(3)
			wound infection (4)	
			transient ischaemic attacks TIA (2)	
– Grade 3	11 (20.4)	4 (15.4)	small or large bowel fistula (3)	surgery (2)
			endoperitoneal bleeding (2)	surgery (2)
			eventration (1)	surgery
			gastric bleeding (1)	interventional radiology

continue →

continue **Table 10.4**

| Ovary | Other | | | |
Morbidity	No. (%)	No. (%)	Complications (No.)	Treatment
			urinary fistula (1)	interventional radiology
			deep venous thrombosis (1)	interventional radiology
			myocardial infarction (1) (1)	intensive care unit
– Grade 4	3 (5.6)	1 (3.8)	pulmonary embolism (2) myocardial infarction (2)	
Postoperative stay (days)	21.5 (8–93)		25.9 (5–90)	
– Primary cytoreduction	23.3 (9–90)		20.7 (5–65)	
– Secondary cytoreduction	19.9 (8–93)		30.6 (12–90)	

led to the development of thermal intolerance. The only adverse event related to HIPEC was cisplatin toxicity (2 cases) in ovarian carcinomatosis and oxaliplatin toxicity (2 cases) in the other group. The major cisplatin-related renal toxicity was grade 1 (WHO) in 1 patient and grade 2 in another: medical treatment reversed both drug-induced reactions. The oxaliplatin toxicity was grade 1 pancreatitis in both patients with serum elevated enzymes reversed in both cases with somastatin and parenteral nutrition.

Morbidity and mortality

Of the 80 patients treated, 48 (60%) had no complications, 13 (16.2%) had minor complications (grade 2) mainly consisting of pleural effusion and wound infections whereas 15 (18.7%) had grade 3 complications: 10 of these required reoperation, three an interventional radiologic procedure and two ICU readmission. Four patients died of pulmonary embolisms (2) and of myocardial infarction (2) during postoperative course, accounting for an in-hospital mortality of 5% (Table 10.4).

Follow-up and Survival

Assessment at discharge showed that most patients (95%) had a satisfactory performance status (equal to or less than 2). In only 4 cases did the poor general conditions of the patient contraindicate the postoperative systemic chemotherapy foreseen in the study protocol.

No patient was lost at follow-up. Of the 76 patients who survived after the surgical procedure 38 (47.5%) are alive and disease free, 10 (12.5%) are alive with disease, 22 (27.5%) died of disease-related causes and 4 (5%) died for causes unrelated to cancer. Mean survival for the ovarian carcinomatosis group was 28.2 months (median 23.5), whereas it was 23.5 months (median 17) in the other group.

The overall 5-year survival was 18.6% in ovarian carcinomatosis and 13.3% in the other group (Figs. 10.2, 10.3). In both groups the survival analysis showed significantly different distribution curves according the CC score (p <0.01 for ovarian carcinomatosis and p <0.003 for others, by log-rank test; Figs. 10.4, 10.5). In the multivariate analysis the Cox proportional-hazard model used to test the simultaneous effect on survival of primary and secondary surgical cytoreduction, CC score and PCI score, the only prognostic factor capable of independently influencing survival was the CC score (p <0.002 for ovarian carcinomatosis, p <0.01 for others; Table 10.5).

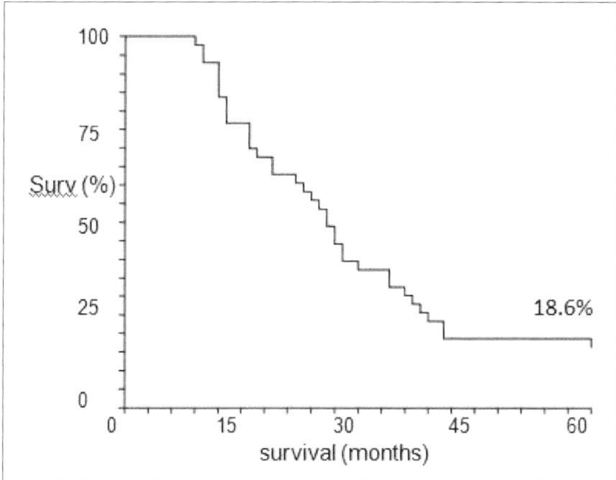

Fig. 10.2 Overall 5-year survival for ovarian carcinomatosis

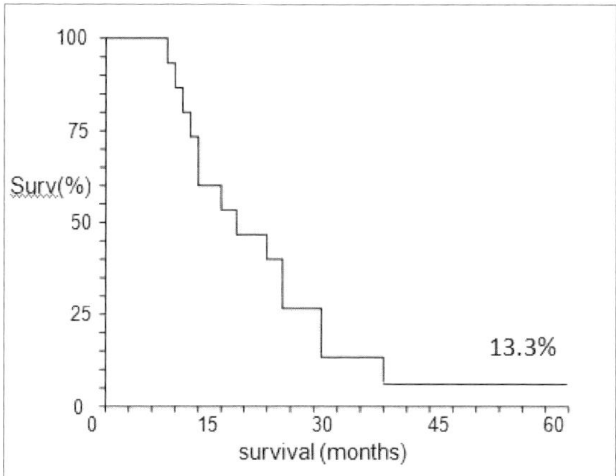

Fig. 10.3 Overall 5-year survival for other malignancy carcinomatosis

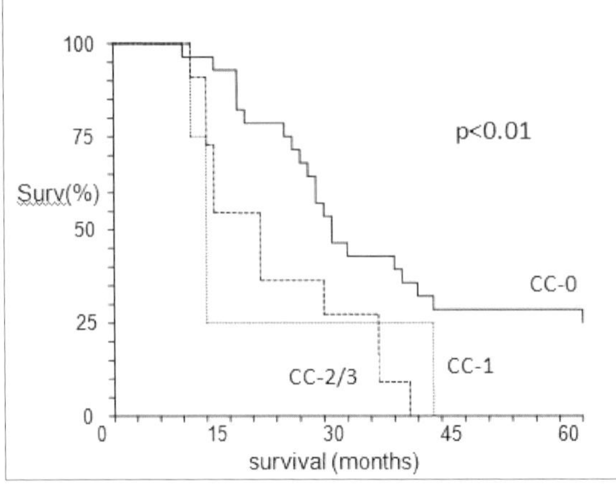

Fig. 10.4 Survival and CC-score for ovarian carcinomatosis

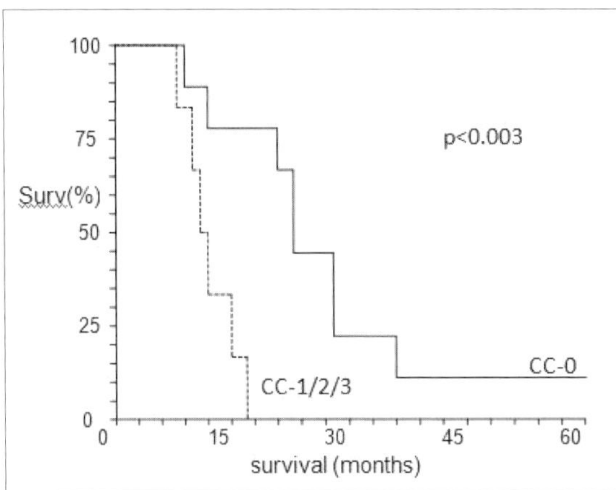

Fig. 10.5 Survival and CC-score for other malignancy carcinomatosis

Table 10.5 Cox regression model of prognostic factors and survival

Variable	Deviance (chi-square)		p	
	Ovary	Other	Ovary	Other
Primary/secondary cytoreduction	3.5455	0.0891	n.s.	n.s.
CC-score	9.2030	5.7964	0.002	0.01
PCI	0.8504	0.0889	n.s.	n.s.

Discussion

Peritoneal carcinomatosis (PC) is one of the most common causes of incurability of intra-abdominal cancers. Surgery or chemotherapy alone are not able to cure these patients. Despite the favorable survival data of CRS and PIC for PSM compared with systemic chemotherapy in the current literature, there are large variations in survival, morbidity and mortality rates across trials and the results should be interpreted with caution for several reasons.

The analysis of the results must bear in mind the different tumors at the basis of the peritoneal diffusion. Better results can be obtained in appendicular tumors (pseudomyxoma peritonei) in ovarian and colorectal carcinomatosis and in mesothelioma, whereas disappointing results have been observed in gastric carcinomatosis and sarcomatosis. In our experience ovarian carcinomatosis accounts for more than half of the cases treated. In agreement with other investigators [28], considering the high recurrence rates after standard treatment for advanced ovarian cancer, and the good results the combined procedures achieved in our series, we suggest that maximal cytoreduction (peritonectomy procedures) plus HIPEC should now be the up-front treatment for selected patients with ovarian carcinomatosis who have diffuse peritoneal spread. Furthermore in this tumor the volume of peritoneal disease (PCI) acquires a less significant prognostic impact in respect to the level of the cytoreduction obtained (CCS), thus justifying surgical efforts even in advanced patients.

A common issue in the combined approach to PSM is to keep the rate of morbidity and mortality of these aggressive treatments under control. The survival benefit is achieved at the expense of moderate morbidity and mortality rates, especially at treatment centers overcoming their initial learning curve, and is dependent on the skills and the level of experience of the surgeon. The results achieved by international experts in this field may not be replicated in routine clinical practice. Overall our patients underwent a total 458 surgical procedures, with a mean 6.3 per case for ovarian carcinomatosis and 4.5 for the other group, a mean duration for the whole procedure (peritonectomy procedures and HIPEC) of 506 minutes and a mean blood loss not exceeding 1950 mL. Considering these data, the number of major complications and operative mortality rate is reasonably low and comes within the range reported by other investigators [13]. The most frequent major complications (Grade 3) were intestinal fistulas owing to the large number of multiple intestinal resections required, bowel-wall weakening during maneuvers to destroy malignant implants in situ, and in our series the increased risk of applying closed HIPEC after completing surgery and after anastomoses had been performed. Whether a fistula is treated conservatively or repaired surgically depends on its quality and volume.

In about 20% of the patients in our series who had minor complications (Grade 2) these were accounted for almost exclusively by wound infections or pleural effusions, events which were particularly frequent in patients who underwent diaphragmatic peritonectomy procedures.

In our surgical series four patients died during the postoperative course, two on day 2, one on day 3 and the fourth on day 5, due to massive pulmonary embolisms and myocardial infarction. The risk of these complications developing is high even despite routine preventive treatment. Notwithstanding prevention, the extent of pelvic resection and the lengthy procedure pose a real risk that is strategically difficult to overcome. Most of our patients had a long postoperative course (about 20 days) and the duration correlated with extent of surgical resection. Conversely, the relatively short mean ICU stay provided evidence that strict patient selection and the proper surgical and anesthetic techniques can keep the procedure-related risks within acceptable limits. Here we underline the importance of having an experienced operating team.

This issue underlines the need for strict selection criteria and a preoperative diagnostic technique able to indicate ideal candidates in whom we can expect the better prognostic results with lower rates of complications. Currently we are very far from this goal. A recent report by Sugarbaker on failure analysis of recurrent disease following complete cytoreduction and PIC in patients with PC from colorectal cancer notes that of 156 selected patients who underwent attempted CRS, complete CRS was possible in only 70 (45%). Furthermore despite the accomplishment of complete cytoreduction, 78% ultimately developed recurrent disease [29]. Clearly better defined criteria for patient selection are needed and this also raises questions about the role of tumor histology and the potential utility of using DNA or protein arrays to determine the genetic signature of the tumor. In addition, it raises concerns as to the potential impact of "neoadjuvant" systemic therapy based on the newer chemotherapy regimens [30].

The technical guidelines for the various types of peritonectomy procedures have been well standardized by Sugarbaker [9–11], but our personal experience suggests a number of considerations. We underline that standardized procedures are easier to apply to primary rather than to secondary cytoreduction. In a patient with a recurrent tumor with PC, planning resection depends crucially on previous surgical procedures. The pelvic peritonectomy procedure proposed by Sugarbaker and used in this series combines en bloc removal of the female reproductive organs, the pouch of Douglas and the rectum, with a complete abdominal pelvic peritonectomy that we always extend to the transverse umbilical line. For several reasons, we rarely restored intestinal continuity with a rectal stump immediately during peritonectomy procedures and HIPEC. Because many of our patients presented with intestinal subocclusion, thus precluding proper preoperative large bowel preparation, we had to limit the development of complications in patients who had undergone especially aggressive interventions, often entailing numerous anastomoses and in whom the protocol envisaged HIPEC. In addition, because the pelvis is the main site of malignant recurrence we preferred to opt for a terminal colostomy in the iliac fossa and postpone restoring intestinal continuity for a second look. In most patients we waited at least 6 months after postperitonectomy systemic chemotherapy before restoring intestinal continuity. In 21 patients in our series extensive large bowel carcinomatosis necessitated a total colectomy, insofar as destroying implants in situ or simply resecting them from the colic wall would have exposed patients to the risk of bowel perforation. Nevertheless, in some cases when technically feasible, total colectomy can be avoided, thus sparing the left transverse colon, left colic flexure and a small portion of the descending colon so that the patient can have a colostomy rather than the poorly tolerated terminal ileostomy.

An especially important point concerns deciding on the best strategy for treating the small bowel, apart from the rectum, which is the intestinal tract most severely involved by carcinomatosis. The number of resections and the extension of resection need careful thought to limit functional damage and allow adequate debulking. Ileal tracts less severely involved by the malignancy are more amenable to in situ treatment. Resecting a nodule is nevertheless often a difficult task owing to deep-seated nodular carcinomatosis disease and to the location, especially if the first jejunal loop is involved or the nodule involves the intestinal wall at the ileo-mesenteric junction. After in situ treatment whenever the wall appears too weak one has to meticulously use interrupted sutures or small patch resections. In situ destruction of mesenteric implants must be meticulous and should continue from the first loop to the ileocecal valve and be followed by a detailed evaluation and treatment first of one, then of the other, mesenteric surface. In most patients in this series extensive tumor spread necessitated upper abdominal procedures to obtain optimal debulking with no visible residual disease. Debulking surgery should in all cases envisage complete greater omentectomy, a key surgical strategy for this disease. In all the patients in this series whom we operated on for recurrence with PC for ovarian cancer and who had undergone surgery elsewhere, laparotomy disclosed carcinomatosis in the residual omentum. Hence omentectomy should envisage removing the entire gastroepiploic arch and skeletalizing the great gastric curve.

Precisely when CRS should include removal of the spleen remains unclear. Although numerous investigators use splenectomy during CRS in a variable percentage of cases none of them specify the criteria for splenectomy [31]. In our experience, apart from patients with evident tumor implants directly involving the spleen, we undertook splenectomy whenever macroscopic malignant implants involved the gastrosplenic ligament. In these cases lymphnode metastases are frequently discovered in the splenic hilum. In our patients with malignant spread to the diaphragmatic peritoneum, a small number of scattered implants were ablated with an argon beam coagulator, electrovaporization, or radiofrequency technology (tissue link). Bulky diaphragmatic disease as well as confluent implants involving an extensive area were usually removed by stripping the peritoneum from the muscle (upper quadrant peritonectomy). This procedure often comprised removing the diseased Glisson capsule, the falciform ligament and hepatic suspensor ligaments. Cholecystectomy was unavoidable also in the presence of small superficial nodules. The presence of even small implants requires the dissection of the hepatoduodenal ligaments and removal of the lesser omentum because destroying even small implants in situ would compromise the integrity of the structures making up the hepatic ligament. Surface pancreatic implants are relatively rare and small nodules can be treated by in situ ablation or excision. Although some studies describe liver resection for metastatic disease in highly selected cases of PC, according to others the presence of liver metastases does not seem sufficient per se to contraindicate CRS [32, 33]. Three patients in our series underwent hepatic resection for metastasis. One of these patients with ovarian carcinomatosis had a major hepatic resection (left hepatic lobectomy) associated with CRS and PIC with an excellent outcome: the patient is alive and has been disease-free for 89 months.

A final technical point concerns the problem of lymph node spread. In our series of ovarian carcinomatosis we routinely removed pelvic and para-aortic lymph nodes in all patients who underwent primary cytoreduction and in many patients who had secondary cytoreduction. An analysis of the site of nodal metastasis nonetheless shows how diffuse peritoneal spread of ovarian malignancy favors extensive lymph node diffusion spreading well beyond the regional drainage to involve the colic and mesorectal lymphnodes at the root of the inferior mesenteric artery, splenic hilum and meso-ileal lymphnodes. Most patients who had metastases in ovarian carcinomatosis had them in extra-regional sites with or without associated regional nodes.

A last important point is the procedure used for HIPEC. Which of the various correctly used procedures is the best – the closed, open, or peritoneal cavity expander technique – remains unclear [34]. Like other investigators [35, 36] we used the closed technique because apart from being safer for staff than the other techniques it makes it easier to achieve a high perfusion temperature. In addition, the higher intra-abdominal pressure reached might increase convection-driven penetration of macromolecular agents inside the tumor and enhance tissue uptake of some chemotherapies [37]. In particular we recommend using amply fenestrated catheters at least 30 cm in length. The spiral drain catheters we use have this characteristic and can be left in situ to save the peritoneal cavity during the postoperative course. In evaluating the overall results of HIPEC we consider it worth mentioning that even in patients in whom surgery achieved suboptimal cytoreduction, HIPEC had the notable benefit of reducing ascites, when present, as others have observed [38] and permitted a better quality of life than in patients treated with traditional methods.

The results we obtained in this series compare well with those of published series especially considering that our patients all had widespread carcinomatosis. We had low mortality and morbidity rates for patients undergoing multiple surgical procedures and HIPEC. Another encouraging finding was that 90% of the patients we treated were able to undergo a further course of systemic chemotherapy within 60 days after surgery. When we analyzed our long-term results, the survival analysis showed that the overall 5-year survival was 18.6% for ovarian carcinomatosis and 13.3% for the other group. These values are both significantly better when we analyze patients with complete cytoreduction. Mean survival was 28.2 months (median 23.5 months) and 23.5 months (median 17), respectively, for the two groups. These survival results are comparable with those reported in the literature considering the high mean PCI values in the ovarian group and the presence of sarcomatoses and gastric carcinomatoses, notably encumbered with a worse prognosis, in the other group.

Conclusions

Our results and the analysis of current literature suggest that CRS plus PIC for selected patients with PC is associated with improved survival when viewed against the prognosis associated with treatment by systemic chemotherapy. Further studies addressing the identification of more stringent selection criteria for patients with PC undergoing the combined approach (CRS plus PIC) can allow the improvement of long-term results in the future. The role of neoadjuvant systemic chemotherapy before primary cytoreduction remains to be investigated in prospective trials.

Acknowledgements
The authors acknowledge the "Azienda Policlinico Umberto I" and "Eleonora Lorillard Spencer Cenci Foundation" for financial support and "B.T. Medical s.r.l." for technical assistance.

References

1. Sugarbaker PH (1994) Pseudomyxoma peritonei. A cancer whose biology is characterized by a redistribution phenomenon Ann Surg 219:109–111
2. Yan TD, Black D, Savady R et al (2006) A systematic review on the efficacy of cytoreductive surgery and perioperative intraperitoneal chemotherapy for pseudomyxoma peritonei. Ann Surg Oncol 14:484–492
3. Ghelen O, Kwiatowsky F, Sugarbaker P.H. et al. Cytoreductive surgery combined with perioperative intraperineal chemotherapy for the management of peritoneal carcinomatosis for colorectal cancer: a multi–istitutional study. J Clin Oncol; 2004, 22:3284–3292
4. Di Giorgio A, Naticchioni E, Biacchi D et al (2008) Cytoreductive surgery (peritonectomy procedures) combined with hipertermic intraperitoneal chemotherapy (HIPEC) in the treatment of diffuse peritoneal carcinomatosis from ovarian cancer. Cancer 113:315–325
5. Yan TD, Brun EA, Cerruto CA et al (2006) Prognostic indicators for patients undergoing cytoreductive surgery and perioperative intraperitoneal chemotherapy for diffuse malignant peritoneal mesotelioma. Ann Surg Oncol 14:41–49
6. Esquivel J (2005) Multidisciplinary sequencial therapy for the treatment of peritoneal surface malignancy of colorectal origin: a plea for cooperation between medical and surgical oncologists. Ann Surg Oncol 12:950–951
7. Sugarbaker PH, Hughes KA (1993) Surgery for colorectal metastasis to liver. In: Wanebo H (ed) Colorectal cancer. Mosby–Year Book, St. Louis, pp 405–413
8.   Sugarbaker PH (1996) Peritoneal carcinomatosis: principle of management. Kluwer, Boston
9. Sugarbaker PH (1995) Peritonectomy procedures. Ann Surg 221:29–42
10. De Lima Vasquez V, Sugarbaker PH (2003) Total anterior parietal peritonectomy. J Surg Oncol 83:261–263
11. De Lima Vasquez V, Sugarbaker PH (2003) Cholecystectomy lesser omentectomy and stripping of the omental bursa: a peritonectomy procedure. J Surg Oncol 84:45–49
12. Elias DM, Ouellet JF (2001) Intraperitoneal chemohyperthermia. Rationale, technique, indications and results. Surg Oncol Clin N Am 10:915–933
13. Yan TD, Zappa L, Edwards G et al (2007) Perioperative outcomes of cytoreductive surgery and perioperative intraperitoneal chemotherapy for non–appendiceal peritoneal carcinomatosis from a prospective database. J Surg Oncol 96:102–112
14. Kusamura S, Younan R, Baratti D et al (2006) Cytoreductive surgery followed by intraperi-

toneal hyperthermic perfusion. Cancer 106:1144–1153

15. Jacquet P, Sugarbaker PH (1996) Clinical research methodologies in diagnosis and staging of patients with peritoneal carcinomatosis. In: Sugarbaker PH (ed) Peritoneal carcinomatosis: principle of management. Kluwer Academic, Boston, pp 359–374

16. Elias D, Blot F, El Otmany A et al (2001) Curative treatment of peritoneal carcinomatosis arising from colorectal cancer by complete resection and intraperitoneal chemotherapy. Cancer 92:71–76

17. Gomes Da Silva R, Sugarbaker PH (2006) Analysis of prognostic factors in seventy patients having a complete cytoreduction plus perioperative intraperitoneal chemotherapy for carcinomatosis from colorectal cancer. J Am Coll Surg 203:878–886

18. Yan TD (2006) Preoperative workup. Proceedings of the 5th International Workshop on Peritoneal Surface Malignancy: December, 4th–6th 2006, Milan, pp 7–8

19. Ronett BM, Yan H, Kurman RJ et al (2001) Patients with pseudomyxoma peritonei associated with disseminated peritoneal adenomucinosis have a significantly more favorable prognosis than patients with peritoneal mucinous carcinomatosis. Cancer 92:85–91

20. Raspagliesi F, Kusamura S, Campos Torres JC et al (2006) Cytoreduction combined with intraperitoneal hyperthermic perfusion chemotherapy in advanced/recurrent ovarian cancer patients: the experience of a National Cancer Institute of Milan. Eur J Surg Oncol 32:671–675

21. Cotte E, Glehen O, Mohamed F et al (2007) Citoreductive surgery and intraperitoneal chemohyperthermia for chemoresistant and recurrent advanced epithelial ovarian cancer: prospective study of 81 patients. World J Surg 31:1813–1820

22. Yan TD, Black D, Savady R et al (2006) Sistematic review on the efficacy of cytoreductive surgery combined with perioperative intraperitoneal chemotherapy for peritoneal carcinomatosis from colorectal carcinoma. J Clin Oncol 24:4011–4018

23. Elias D, Raynard B, Farkhondeh F et al (2006) Peritoneal carcinomatosis of colorectal origin: long–term results of intraperitoneal chemohyperthermia with oxaliplatin following complete cytoreductive surgery. Gastroenterol Clin Biol 30:1200–1204

24. Verwaal VJ, Van Ruth S, De Bree E et al (2003) Randomized trial of cytoreduction and hyperthermic intraperitoneal chemotherapy versus systemic chemotherapy and palliative surgery in patients with peritoneal carcinomatosis of colorectal cancer. J Clin Oncol 21:3737–3743

25. Esquivel J, Sticca R, Sugarbaker PH et al (2006) Cytoreductive surgery and hyperthermic intraperitoneal chemotherapy in the management of peritoneal surface malignancies of colonic origin: a consensus statement. Ann Surg Oncol 14:128–133

26. World Health Organization (1979) WHO handbook for reporting results of cancer treatment. WHO, Geneva

27. Bozzetti F, Braga M, Gianotti L et al (2001) Postoperative enteral versus parenteral nutrition in malnourished patients with gastrointestinal cancer: randomized multicentre trial. Lancet 358:1487–1492

28. Reichman TW, Cracchiolo B, Sama J et al (2005) Cytoreductive surgery and intraoperative hyperthermic chemoperfusion for advanced ovarian carcinoma. J Surg Oncol 90:56–58

29. Bijelic L, Yan TD, Sugarbaker PH (2007) Failure analysis of recurrent disease following complete cytoreduction and perioperative intraperitoneal chemotherapy in patients with peritoneal carcinomatosis from colorectal cancer. Ann Surg Oncol 14:2281–2288

30. Lambert LA, Mansfield PF (2007) Cytoreductive surgery and perioperative peritoneal chemotherapy for colorectal carcinomatosis: if at first you don't succeed... Ann Surg Oncol 14:3037–3039

31. Magtibay PM, Adams PB, Silverman MB et al (2006) Splenectomy as part of cytoreductive surgery in ovarian cancer. Gynecol Oncol 102:369–374

32. Merideth MA, Cliby WA, Keeney GL et al (2003) Hepatic resection for metachronous metastases from ovarian carcinoma. Gynecol Oncol 89:16–21

33. Kianmanesh R, Scaringi S, Sabate JM et al (2007) Iterative cytoreductive surgery associated with hyperthermic intraperitoneal chemotherapy for treatment of peritoneal carcinomato-

sis of colorectal origin with or without liver metastases. Ann Surg 245:597–603
34. Glehen O (2006) Hyperthermic intraoperative chemotherapy: nomenclature and modality of perfusion. Proceedings of the 5th International Workshop on Peritoneal Surface Malignancy: December, 4th–6th 2006, Milan, pp 17–18
35. Loggie BV, Fleming RA, Mc Quellon RP et al (2000) Cytoreductive surgery with intraperitoneal hyperthermic chemotherapy for disseminated cancer of gastrointestinal origin. Am Surg 66:561–568
36. Glehen O, Cotte E, Schreiber V et al (2004) Intraperitoneal chemohyperthermia and attempted cytoreductive surgery in patients with peritoneal carcinomatosis of colorectal origin. Br J Surg 91:747–754
37. Milosevic MF, Fyles AV, Hill RP et al (1999) The relationship between elevated interstitial fluid pressure and blood flow in tumors: a bioengineering analysis. Int J Radiat Oncol Biol Phys 44:1111–1123
38. Deraco M, Rossi CR, Pennacchioli E et al (2001) Cytoreductive surgery followed by intraperitoneal hyperthermic perfusion in the treatment of recurrent epithelial ovarian cancer: a phase II clinical study. Tumori 87:120–126

Chapter 11

Pelvic Recurrences of Rectal Cancer

Antonio Bolognese, Luciano Izzo, Pierfrancesco Di Cello, Dario Pietrasanta, Alessandro Crocetti, Silvia Trombetta

Local-regional recurrences (LRRs) after curative surgery for rectal cancer are one of the major problems of colorectal surgery. In fact, despite the significant improvements of preoperative methods to verify the stage of the disease, the introduction of neoadjuvant radiochemotherapy and the enhancement of the surgical technique, a substantial number of patients experience a recurrence. The adoption of a valid follow-up protocol enables the early diagnosis of the presence of recurrences, thus increasing the chance of recovery.

The pelvis is the most frequent site of local recurrences of disease and has a high curative potentiality. Every year in the United States there are an estimated 36,000–38,000 new cases of rectal cancer [1]. In Italy there are an estimated 25,000–30,000 new cases each year. After curative surgery, a recurrence may occur in up to 40% of these cases [2], usually within the first two years after surgery. The percentage survival of patients with local recurrence that cannot be resected is less than 4% at 5 years [3]. More than 50% of these patients are carriers of a recurrence than can be removed by surgery, the only potentially curative therapeutic action, with minimum mortality and an estimated five-year survival rate around 30% [3, 4].

It has been suggested that LRRs are one of the major problems of colorectal surgery and often a surgical unknown factor; this is based on the fact that the diagnosis is often very difficult and that surgical treatment is rarely radical [5].

Various studies have reported an incidence of LRRs between 3 and 30% [6, 7]. This wide range is to be ascribed to different guidelines in the primary treatment of rectal cancer, which is still not homogeneously treated in relation to the total mesorectal excision (TME) technique [8], to the extension of the pelvic lateral lymphadenectomy [9], and to the combination of complementary radiochemotherapies [10].

In 90% of cases LRRs occur within the first 2 years after surgery, rarely after 5 years [3, 5]. The percentage rate and onset of LRRs are correlated to a number of anatomosurgical and biologic factors which influence the risk of their formation.

Chiotasso [11] was one of the first to identify a higher rate of recurrences in distal rectal cancer, both because of the complete absence of the mesorectum at

A. Bolognese, L. Izzo (eds.), *Surgery in Multimodal Management of Solid Tumors.*
©Springer-Verlag Italia 2009

that site, resulting in a higher extension of the tumor, and because of the different lymphatic diffusion (Table 11.1). Among the biological factors, the same prognostic factors impacting the survival rate determine the risk of recurrence: the more advanced the Dukes stage, the higher the risk. Other prognostic factors and additional risk factors are reported in Table 11.2 and mainly regard the presence or absence of lymphatic, venous or perineural invasion and molecular markers [12–20].

As for LRR pathogenesis, a distinction needs to be made between cases of persistence of disease and cases of a real reoccurrence of the disease after curative resection, i.e. LRR.

Quirke reported some cases in 1986 in 'Lancet' [21] and later in 2007 [22] in which a thorough study of the resected part showed some residues of neoplastic cells in the surrounding tissues, defining them as cases with persistence of the disease, with a clearly unfavorable prognosis. Real LRRs after curative resection are instead mostly related to neoplastic micro-foci not included in the exeresis or to metastases of exfoliated tumor cells or to metachronous carcinogenesis, considering that pure anastomotic recurrences are rare [22–24].

Table 11.1 Particularity of lower rectal cancer [11]

	Proximal rectum	Distal rectum
Lymph node invasion	31.3 %	7.8%
Distal intramural extension	21.9 %	11.0 %
Pelvic recurrence	22.0 %	11.0 %

Table 11.2 Tumor recurrence and prognostic factors [13]

Relapses are more frequent for sub-peritoneal rectum, and the most significant prognostic factor is tumor stage	
Dukes A	2–3 %
Dukes B	About 20 %
Dukes C	About 50%
Other prognostic factors	*Risk factors*
CEA	Stage*
Age	Embolic or lymphatic, venous and perineural invasion
Histologic type	Aneuploid DNA
Perforation	High preoperative CEA
Occlusion	Young age
Manipulation	Type of surgery
	Resection extension
	Immune status
	Clinical anastomotic leak

*Tumor infiltrating the perirectal fat ≤6 mm → 5% incidence of LRRs versus 20% for major infiltrations

In about 50% of cases, LRRs are found exclusively in the pelvis, with no distant metastases [4], and as such they can be subjected to surgery with curative intent, with a technique increasingly more aggressive than in the past.

Higher possibilities of curative treatment are related to a very early diagnosis of LRRs. The challenge, therefore, is achieving this early diagnosis to allow the highest chance of cure. Although most surgeons recommend monitoring after resection, there is no agreement about the frequency of follow-up and diagnostic modalities. Diagnosis is frequently clinical (Table 11.3) and pain is the most frequent symptom, and may be abdominal, pelvic, perineural and sometimes sciatic.

The clinical examination is based on abdominal palpation, rectal and vaginal exploration and on palpation of lymph node stations. The invasion of the intestinal lumen by the recurrence after anterior resection causes rectal bleeding and alvine alterations.

Instrumental diagnosis is based on laboratory tests, endoscopic evaluation and on the most up-to-date imaging diagnosis.

In order to define a recurrence prior to surgery, the international literature reports several classifications based on a number of the characteristics of recurrences, with adhesiveness to one or more sites and invasion of the adjacent organs being particularly important [5, 25] (Table 11.4), given the consequent contraindications to surgical resection. In particular, the presence of disease external to the pelvis represents a contraindication to reoperation, except in the presence of completely resectable liver and/or pulmonary metastasis, as well as in the case of invasion of the sacrum above the S2–S3 articulation.

Table 11.3 Diagnosis of LRRs [3]

Clinical examination

Diagnosis is frequently clinical with pain being the most frequent symptom

Clinical examination is based on abdominal palpation, rectal and vaginal exploration and on palpation of lymph nodes

70% of patients with LRRs after anterior resection present a palpable mass

Laboratory tests: CEA

↑ especially in case of liver metastasis

Negative in 50% of LRRs

Instrumental tests

Trans-rectal or trans-vaginal US

Endoscopy

CT scan

MR scan (particularly useful to solve differences between recurrences and fibrous tissue)

RIGS

PET scan (not easily accessible – very expensive)

Table 11.4 Tumor recurrence characteristics and T-stage

Recurrence characteristics [5]		
F0	No adhesion	34.4 %
F1	Adhesion to one site	43.7 %
F2	Adhesion to two or more sites	21.9 %
T-stage (Wanebo classification [24])		
Tr1-2	invasion in bowel wall (subserosal)	
Tr3	invasion in perirectal fat	
Tr4	invasion in anterior urogenital organs	
Tr5	invasion of sacrum or pelvic side walls	

Treatment of rectal carcinoma recurrence is necessarily multimodal [10]. Therapy is based on preoperative radiochemotherapy (except in patients previously irradiated for treatment of the primary disease), followed by surgical resection and often by adjuvant chemotherapy.

LRR surgical treatment can be either radical or palliative and ranges from a simple perineal or vaginal excision to partial or total pelvectomy with, when possible, reconstructive sacral and plastic resections for the closure of the perineal rupture. Surgical treatment, however, should tend to R0 curative resections, which have an acceptable mortality rate with satisfactory long-term survival. Some studies report 80% recurrence rates with 35% curability and 20–30% 5-year survival with 50-70% total control of the disease.

Furthermore, it can be assumed that there is a space for palliative type surgery (R1-R2), provided it enables a higher survival rate to be attained and an improvement in the quality of life of these patients (Table 11.5) [22, 26–29].

Table 11.5 Survival [27, 28]

Exeresis	No. of patients	3 years	5 years
R0	65	57 %	38 %
R1	11	44 %	27 %
R2	95	26 %	15 %

Institutional Experience

In order to evaluate the incidence of LRR in our personal experience, we retrospectively reviewed the clinical charts of all patients treated for rectal cancer at "Pietro Valdoni" Surgery Department from 1998 to 2007.

Population and Perioperative Work-up

During this 10 year period we observed a total of 368 patients with a diagnosis of primary rectal cancer (Table 10.6).

All patients were adequately staged preoperatively by means of colonoscopy, total body CT scan and abdominal ultrasonography. Oncologic markers such as CEA and CA19-9 were also evaluated. Especially during the last 5 years, patient workup has generally included MR of the pelvis and endorectal ultrasonography, which has proven to be very effective for the preoperative evaluation of cancer extension (T parameter) and the presence and extension of lymph node involvement (N parameter).

Table 11.6 Institutional experience 1998/2007 "P. Valdoni" surgery department

	Total	Male	Female	Rate (%)
Patients	368	232	136	100.0
Distal rectum	102	58	44	27.7
Middle rectum	119	77	42	32.3
Proximal rectum	103	73	30	28.0
Junction	31	18	13	8.4
Not available	13			3.5

General and Surgical Management

Of the 368 identified patients, 7 were judged not amenable to any surgical management, either because of the extension of the disease or due to advanced age and/or poor general conditions. Forty-eight patients underwent palliative surgical treatment, mainly to avoid or solve an intestinal occlusion, and consisting either of the creation of a colostomy (22 cases), the placing of an endoprothesis (3 patients) or a Hartmann intervention (23 patients).

In total, 288 patients underwent a surgical procedure with curative intent. In most cases the type of surgery was either ARR (211 cases) or Miles intervention (52 cases). In all cases, a total mesorectal excision (TME) was performed, according to the international protocols. In 15 cases the neoplasm was excised through a TEM procedure, while in 4 cases a trans-anal excision was performed; in 3 cases the surgeon decided to perform a total colectomy (due either to poor blood supply or to multiple colonic perforations), and in 3 patients diagnosis of rectal cancer was achieved through an endoscopic polipectomy, and no more procedures were performed because the neoplasm was totally excised (Tables 10.7, 10.8). Morbidity and mortality are reported in Table 10.9.

Table 11.7 Surgical management of primary cancer

No Surgery	**7**	**1.90 %**
Palliative Surgery	**48**	**13.00 %**
Colostomy	22	
Endoprosthesis	3	
Hartmann	23	
Neoadjuvant Chemoradiation	**75**	**20.40 %**
Proximal rectum	7	
Middle rectum	26	
Distal rectum	41	
Junction	1	
Curative Surgery	**288**	**78.26 %**

Table 11.8 Curative management of primary cancer

Anterior Rectal Resection	**211**	**73.26 %**
Tis/T1	27	
T2	43	
T3	130	
T4	11	
Proximal rectum	92	
Middle rectum	73	
Distal rectum	27	(Colo-anal anastomosis: 13 cases)
Junction	19	
Miles operation	**52**	**18.00 %**
Tis/T1	3	
T2	14	
T3	34	
T4	1	
TEM	**15**	**4.00 %**
Others	**10**	**2.70 %**

Table 11.9 Morbidity/mortality

Perioperative mortality	**3.48 %**
Perioperative morbidity	**12.50 %**
Anastomosis leaks/fistulae	26 cases
Pelvic abscess	3 cases
Surgical wound leak	3 cases
Perioperative bleeding	2 cases

Local-Regional Recurrences: Incidence and Patient Work-up

Of these 288 patients, 31 (11%) showed an LRR. We also treated 11 patients previously managed elsewhere for the primary cancer; thus, we managed in total 42 patients with LRR. There were 26 males and 16 females, with a M/F ratio of 1.62. Their age ranged from 37 to 86 years, with a mean age of 65.8. We decided to focus on the 35 patients who showed no distant metastases at the time of the previous surgical treatment (Table 10.10).

Table 11.10 Local-regional occurrences

LRR (no./rate)	32	11 %
Total managed patients	42	
M/F ratio	1.62	
Mean age	65.8	(range 37–86)
Absence of distal metastasis at former surgery	35	

Primary rectal cancer was T4 in 9 cases (25.7%), T3 in 18 cases (51.4%), T2 in 7 cases (20%) and T1 in 1 case (2.8%). Former surgical treatment was ARR in 21 cases (60%), Miles intervention in 9 cases (25.7%), Hartmann procedure in 4 cases (11.4%) and TEM in 1 case (2.8%). In 31 cases (88.5%) the resection score had been assessed as R0, while it had been assessed as R1-R2 in 4 cases (11.5%). In 6 patients (17.1%) a neoadjuvant chemoradiation therapy had been administered, while 20 patients (57.1%) underwent adjuvant chemoradiation therapy after surgical management.

As for the site of recurrence, LRR were stratified as follows: 13 (37.1%) anastomotic recurrences, 11 centro-pelvic recurrences (31.4%), 9 pre-sacral recurrences (25.7%) and 2 perineal recurrences (5.7%). Involved organs were most commonly ureters, bladder, sacrum and pelvic bones, while no involvement of the sciatic nerve or iliac vessels was documented. LRR presented with abdominal pain in 27 patients (77.1%), with palpable abdominal mass in 16 patients (45.7%), and/or with an increase in the value of blood oncologic markers in 12 patients (34.3%).

Disease-Free Survival (DFS) ranged from 3 to 51 months from surgery, with a mean value of 13.4. Patient workup included blood exams (with oncologic markers), colonoscopy, abdominal, endorectal and transvaginal US, total body CT scan and MR scan. Neoadjuvant chemoradiation therapy was performed in 12 patients (42.8%). Patient stratification is summarized in Table 11.11.

Local-Regional Recurrences: General and Surgical Management

Seven patients were judged not amenable to surgical treatment, because of the presence of diffuse lung or liver metastases (4 patients), or due to infiltration of the sacrum or pelvic bones.

Table 11.11 Patient stratification (35 cases)

Former treatment		
ARR	21	60.0%
Miles	9	25.7%
Hartmann	4	11.4%
TEM	1	2.8%
Former resection score		
R0	31	88. 6%
R1–R2	4	11.4%
Primary rectal cancer		
T1	1	2.8%
T2	7	20.0%
T3	18	51.4%
T4	9	25.7%
Dukes A	2	5.7%
Dukes B	6	17.1%
Dukes C	27	77.2%
Site of recurrence		
Anastomotic	13	37.1%
Centro-pelvic	11	31.4%
Pre-sacral	9	25.7%
Perineal	2	5.7%

Surgical management was performed in 28 patients, according to site and extension of recurrent neoplasm and to the patient's general conditions. In 23 cases surgery was performed with curative intent, while for 5 patients palliative surgery was carried out. Potentially curative surgical management included 7 new rectal resections (each of them on previous ARR), 10 recurrent neoplasm exeresis (5 on previous ARR, 4 on previous Miles intervention, 1 on previous Hartmann procedure) and 6 Miles procedures (4 on previous ARR, 1 on previous Hartmann intervention, 1 on previous TEM) (Table 11.12).

Postoperative morbidity was 42.8%, mostly due to anastomotic leak (6 cases), intestinal occlusion (3 cases) and pelvic abscess, peritonitis, thrombosis (1 case each). Two patients (7.1%) died in the postoperative period from cardiac arrest and from hemorrhagic shock, respectively (Table 11.13).

Twenty-three patients (78.5%) subsequently underwent adjuvant chemotherapy. Actual follow-up shows a mean OS of 29.2 months, ranging from 9 to 85 months from LRR diagnosis. In 18 cases (64.2%) the second surgery led to an R0 resection, thus leading to a complete recovery; in 10 cases resection score was assessed as R1-2 and, after a period ranging from 2 to 13 months (mean 5), patients showed recurrence/disease progression.

Table 11.12 LRR management

No surgical treatment	7	**20.0 %**
Palliative treatment	5	**14.3 %**
Curative surgery	23	**65.7 %**
Excision of recurrence	10	
New rectal resection	7	
Miles operation	6	

Table 11.13 LRR morbidity / mortality

Perioperative mortality	**7.1 %**
Cardiac arrest	1 case
Hemorrhagic shock	1 case
Perioperative morbidity	**42.8 %**
Anastomic leaks/fistulae	6 case
Intestinal occlusion	3 case
Pelvic abscess	1 case
Peritonitis	1 case
Thrombosis	1 case

Conclusions

The introduction of TME in common surgical practice and the multimodal therapeutic approach to rectal cancer, managed by an interdisciplinary team of surgeons, oncologists, radiologists and radiotherapists, have led to a dramatic decrease in the incidence of LRR after rectal cancer.

Moreover, as was previously the case with peritoneal carcinosis, LRR are no longer seen as a terminal stage of rectal cancer, and thus excluded from any therapeutic chance, but as a locally advanced disease which, if some conditions are respected (such as absence of distant metastases and absence or potentially resectable involvement of sacrum and pelvis bones), can be amenable to different therapeutic options.

In these selected patients, LRR may be amenable to a multimodal approach which in a significant number of cases can lead to a potentially curative, R0 resection, and in the other cases to palliative management able to improve both overall survival and, above all, the quality of life of these patients.

In particular, our data show a mean OS of more than 2 years after surgical management of a LRR; in more than 64% of cases the second surgery led to a R0 resection, thus leading to a complete recovery, while in the other 36% of patients we achieved our primary goal, consisting of offering a satisfactory quality of life even for R1-R2 patients.

References

1. Bal DG (2001) Cancer Statistics 2001: Quo Vadis or Whither Goes thou? CA Cancer J Clin 51: 11–14
2. Abuafi AM, Williams NS (1994) Local recurrence of colorectal cancer: the problem, mechanisms, management and adjuvant therapy. Br J Surg 81:7–19
3. Maetani S, Onodera H, Nishitani T (2007) Long-term cure in surgery for extrarectal pelvic recurrence of rectal cancer. Dis Colon Rectum 50:1558–1565
4. Garcia-Aguilar J, Cromwell JW, Marra C et al (2001) Treatment of locally recurrent rectal cancer. Dis Colon Rectum 44:1743–1748
5. Boyle KM, Sagar PM, Chalmers AG et al (2005) Surgery for locally recurrent rectal cancer. Dis Colon Rectum 48:929–937
6. Sagar PM, Pemberton JH (1996) Surgical management of locally recurrent rectal cancer. Br J Surg 83:293–304
7. Kapiteijn E, Marijnen CA, Nagtegaal ID et al (2001) Preoperative radiotherapy combined with total mesorectal excision for resectable rectal cancer. N Eng J Med 345:638–646
8. Heald RJ, Husband EM, Ryall MD (1982) The mesorectum in rectal cancer surgery – the clue to pelvic recurrence? Br J Surg 69:613–616
9. Moriya Y, Hojo K, Sawada T, Koyama Y (1989) Significance of lateral node dissection for advanced rectal carcinoma at or below the peritoneal reflection. Dis Colon Rectum 32:307–315
10. Rodel C, Grabenbauer G, Matzel KE et al (2000) Extensive surgery after high-dose preoperative chemioradiotherapy for locally advanced recurrent rectal cancer. Dis Colon Rectum 43:312–319
11. Gamagami RA, Liagre A, Chiotasso P et al (1999) Coloanal anastomosis for distal third rectal cancer: prospective study of oncologic results. Dis Colon Rectum 42:1272–1275
12. Nicholls J (2007) Local excision of rectal carcinoma. Colorectal Dis 9:771–772
13. Goldberg PA, Nicholls RJ (1995) Prediction of local recurrence and survival of carcinoma of the rectum by surgical and histopathological assessment of local clearance. Br J Surg 82:1054–1056
14. Gilbertsen VA (1962) The results of the surgical treatment of cancer of the rectum. Surg Gynecol Obstet 114:313–319
15. Morson BC, Bussey HJ (1967) Surgical pathology of rectal cancer in relation to adjuvant radiotherapy. B J Radiol 40(471):161–165
16. Michelassi F, Block GE, Vannucci L et al (1988) A 5- to 21 years follow-up and analysis of 250 patients with rectal adenocarcinoma. Ann Surg 208:379–389
17. Phillips RKS, Hittinger R, Blesovsky L et al (1984) Local recurrence following "curative" surgery for large bowel cancer II: the rectum and recto-sigmoid. Br J Surg 71:17–20
18. Scott NAS, Rainwater LM, Wieand HS et al (1987) The relative prognostic value of flow cytometric DNA analysis and conventional clinico-pathologic criteria in patients with operable rectal carcinoma. Dis Colon Rectum 30:513–520
19. Hamelin R, Laurent-Puigh P, Olschwang S et al (1994) Association of p-53 mutations with short survival in colorectal cancer. Gastroenterology 106:42–48
20. Lee SI, Kim SH, Wang HM et al (2008) Local recurrence after laparoscopic resection of T3 rectal cancer without preoperative chemoradiation and a risk group analysis: an asian collaborative study. J Gastrointest Surg 12(5):933–938
21. Quirke P, Durdey P, Dixon MF, Willams MF (1986) Local recurrence of rectal adenocarcinoma due to inadequate surgical resection. Histopathological study of lateral tumour spread and surgical excision. Lancet 2(8514):996–999

22. Quirke P, Morris E (2007) Reporting colorectal cancer Histopathology 50:103–112
23. Rosenberg IL, Russell CW, Giles GR (1978) Cell viability studies on the exfoliated colonic cancer cell. Br J Surg 65:188–190
24. Umpleby HC, Fermor B, Symes MO et al (1984) Viability of exsfoliated colorectal carcinoma cells. Br J Surg 71:659–663
25. Wanebo HJ, Antoniuk P, Koness RJ et al (1999) Pelvic resection of recurrent rectal cancer: technical considerations and outcomes. Dis Colon Rectum 42:1438–1448
26. Delpero JR, Lasser P (2000) Curative treatment of local and regional rectal cancer recurrences. Ann Chir 125:818–824
27. Suzuki K, Dozois RR, Devine RM et al (1996) Curative reoperations for locally recurrent rectal cancer. Dis Colon Rectum 39:730–736
28. Radice E, Dozois RR (2001) Locally recurrent rectal cancer. Dig Surg 18:355–362
29. Billiet C, Berard P, Rivoalan F et al (2006) Results of resection of locally recurrent rectal cancer. Ann Chir 131:601–607

Subject Index

Printed in Italy in September 2008